The
Pregnancy
Experience

McKenzie Nelson

Fulton Books
Meadville, PA

Published by Fulton Books 2024

ISBN 979-8-89221-154-3 (paperback)
ISBN 979-8-89221-156-7 (digital)

Printed in the United States of America

To my husband, Chris, thank you for taking this journey with me through the hardest challenge we've ever faced. Thank you for the support, the back rubs, the help with stretches, your kindness, your love, and a million other things.

To the women who were courageous and kind enough to share their birthing stories with me without filter, thank you for helping new moms know what they could potentially expect in this whirlwind of a phase they're going through.

Contents

Author's Note

The beauty about families is every family dynamic is completely different, and I aim to be as inclusive in my writing as possible without having to list ten different roles that could fill the position I'm discussing in the pages of this book. Please note that anytime I use the terms "spouse" or "husband," I really mean whoever is going to be supporting you and your baby at this time in your life. This person could be a friend, parent, grandparent, nanny, doula, husband, wife, partner, sister, brother, or anything in between.

In the interest of brevity, I have used our family dynamic as the basis for this book so I can feel as close to the work as possible. My hope is seeing myself in the memories of the growth and birth of my child as I write will provide me with a deeper connection to the book and will allow the reader the greatest insight into my experience.

I have only had what doctors call a singleton birth, which means I've only ever had one baby at a time, and the wording in this book reflects that as well. Please read the word "baby" as "babies" at any point in this book if you'll be having more than one child at once.

I have a brother with open-back spina bifida, which means as much as I would have loved to have delivered with a midwife, I wasn't trusting my family history to anyone but a doctor. Please replace the word "doctor" with "midwife" or "home-birthing coach" wherever relevant.

This book is meant to help you know what to expect of yourself emotionally and physically in each trimester of pregnancy; therefore, it's very helpful if you read a trimester ahead of where you are in your pregnancy journey so you know what to expect before it happens to you, and you can decide how you'd like to handle/react/avoid it before you're in the moment.

I have excluded the science of what happens to you in each trimester since there are plethora of books that cover those topics already, and I wanted to provide moms to be with something they could read and absorb quickly that hasn't been beaten to death.

Nothing in this book should be used as a replacement for professional help (i.e., doctors, therapists, etc.), but hopefully this book can help ease some of the pain of your journey.

Zeroth Trimester

Deciding to Try through Finding Out You're Pregnant

Pregnancy is *not* a nine-month journey like most people will have you believe. I had heard so many people bring up the nine-month deadline that in my head, I was like "yes, after nine months, I'm done."

No!

Be prepared to embark on *at least* a yearlong journey from conception, and that is at the absolute minimum, for reasons that will be seen in the fourth trimester section. If you decide to breastfeed, you're looking at an even longer journey before you're back to what you'd consider your more "normal self."

The end of the forty weeks is not the end of the battle. Tell yourself that pregnancy is at least a yearlong journey so you don't have your baby and think, *Oh good! I'm done.*

Buckle up, buttercup, the fun is just beginning!

Before you decide you want to have a baby, you and your spouse need to get to a place of openness and emotional maturity together.

You need to be comfortable bringing up uncomfortable topics and getting to the end of those discussions, not fighting and giving up before a resolution is reached, promising you'll go back to it later or fighting, giving up, and never finishing the conversation, inadvertently allowing things to continue as they are.

You will need to rely on your spouse after your baby is born, and you will need to know how to express to them your need for help. You should be in a place where you can make them understand you're not asking for help because you want to do less; you're asking because you're not sure how you're going to keep moving forward without that help.

If you can't bring up everything and anything sex-related to your spouse before you have a kid, your road ahead is going to be harder than it needs to be. When you need to explain to your spouse at 2:00 a.m. that fluid is leaking out of your vagina and you have to change the sheets and potentially go to the hospital, you don't want to be so emotionally stunted with them that you feel embarrassed that your body is reacting this way.

Take prenatal vitamins three months before you start trying for a baby. It's great for the baby and helps protect them from some very preventable conditions, but it's also awesome for your complexion, hair, and nails, so you'll see something in return for you. If your body has been missing something, this can really help level out your moods and make you feel better day-to-day. Some vitamins are only absorbed with food in your system, so try to take your vitamins after eating something to get the full benefits. Most doctors' offices won't see you until you're eight to ten weeks pregnant, so by the time the doctor would tell you to start these, you're basically done the first trimester. Check out appendix 1 for a general idea of what to expect from doctor appointments.

As soon as you decide you'd like to have a baby, that same conversation should involve discussing with your spouse how to split the workload in the house, if you haven't already done so. Sure, you'll need more help when the baby is born, but your first and third trimesters, you'll be exhausted and not be able to do as much as you had been, so set the expectation before you find yourself needing extra help. The added stress of bridging those topics when utterly exhausted with a dump truck full of hormones coursing through your veins is not something I'd wish on anyone. So don't allow yourself to be the main/only person taking care of the house before this begins. Get your spouse used to the idea of splitting the load before it becomes a necessity.

Train your body to drink one hundred ounces of water every day before your bladder gets small. Have it adjust to higher fluid intakes early. You're going to pee *like crazy* at first, but it should help in the end. Drink electrolytes if you get a headache while you're trying to increase your water intake. You can drink enough water that you've diluted the electrolytes in your body, which can present as a headache.

Once you've decided you're ready to start trying to have a baby, it can be incredibly frustrating if you're not pregnant immediately. I was surprised how quickly I became impatient, especially knowing you have such a short window to be successful each month. Concerns that you or your spouse's body can't make a baby properly, or something you did forever ago is affecting you now, pop up very quickly. Remember, it's a process, and don't point fingers at each other to add even more stress. Instead, enjoy the moments together and your last few months of starfishing on the bed after sex…because those don't happen nearly enough when you have a newborn.

If you haven't learned about your period cycle and the times in your cycle when it is easiest to get pregnant, you should do that now. Knowing how your cycle works can increase your chances of becoming pregnant and reduce the amount of time you need to try before conceiving.

Do you have a good support system surrounding you to lean on during your pregnancy and after your baby is born? We're an hour and a half from our closest family and had moved into a new state during COVID-19, so we didn't have close local friends to rely on during my pregnancy, which meant to get help, we needed to wait at least an hour and a half for it to arrive. You're thinking, *No big deal, we're planners, and I don't like people showing up unannounced anyways.* Well, that's all fine and dandy until you unexpectedly have to go to the ER at 6:00 a.m., and your support system then has to fight through morning rush hour traffic to get to you.

Fun fact (at least at our local ER): ERs won't let a three-month-old into the ER or the ER lobby, which means for my three-month postpartum unexpected ER trip, my husband and baby waited for two hours in the car for my mom to show up while I waited in the ER alone, trying to figure out what was wrong with my body. It takes a whole village to raise a child; even if your village is just one other family, it's enough.

Start stretching your hips, working out your lower back muscles, building up muscles in your pelvic floor, working up your biceps, curling fifteen to twenty pounds, and squatting. Make your body feel good before it starts feeling the stress of pregnancy. Most doctors will tell you continuing any workouts you've been doing before pregnancy is fine but that you should not start anything new during pregnancy. The above are all things that will make the pregnancy or postpartum part of your life significantly easier (e.g., strong pelvic floors birth and support babies better, and bicep curling fifteen to twenty pounds is *exactly* what you'll be doing, carrying around a baby and a car seat on *day 2* of your child's birth).

Take a picture of your lady bits. It sounds weird, but if you need stitches from a vaginal birth, all of a sudden, there are a lot of questions about "Is this normal for me?" and "Is this how it should look?" Having something to compare it to helps since every woman is a little different.

Even the most understanding of spouses will end up trying to unknowingly repress you at some point in time. They think they're helping and know what's "best" for all of you, but it doesn't feel like that, and a lot of time, they're giving you advise based on things that are not backed by science, are rooted in their emotions, they saw online, or are outdated myths. *So*

❖ be able to express your emotions without becoming emotional,

❖ have science-based facts to counter untrue arguments (I'd recommend Emily Oster's *Expecting Better* as a good place to start), and

❖ ensure you have *you and your baby's* best interest at heart. Don't get so wrapped up in doing everything you can for the baby that you forget to do things for yourself as well.

Hopefully, this book will help you, but if you're still apprehensive about what you're about to go through, ask other moms you know if they'll share their birth experience with you. In my experience, any mom I've talked to has seemed to want a safe space to talk about what happened to them during the growth and delivery of their baby. You just need to let them know you'd like to hear their story and that they're not overstepping. I've interviewed some moms I know and have included their stories in appendix 2 in case you don't know anyone who has done this recently. The more birthing stories you hear, the more you can be prepared for what your pregnancy and delivery day could look like.

First Trimester

Finding Out You're Pregnant through the Twelfth Week

Learn the parts of your vagina! I went to school in the United States during a time when abstinence was the main form of sex education, and as a result, I was horrified to realize during a nine-month pregnancy appointment that I wasn't positive what every part of my vagina was called.

When I told my male doctor I was having pain in "this part" of my vagina and pointed and he said "in your labia?" I was like "ah, yes, labia, that is a vaginal term" and then realized I wasn't positive the labia was the "lips" and was too embarrassed to admit that or say "the lips." So I just said yes and hoped to God I was right.

Then all I could think for the rest of the night was how embarrassed I was that a man, even though this was his profession, knew more about my body than I did. Why did I never realize how little I had been taught to know about myself because it was an "off-limits" topic in my house? Or because my school decided the best way to teach people not to get pregnant at a young age was through sheer ignorance?

Learn your body! By terminology? Great. By touch? Even better. Things are going to be pretty inflamed for a while after a vaginal delivery, so knowing what was "normal" helps.

Remember, this is your own experience, and your feelings are valid. No one gets to tell you how to be a parent or tell you that what you're feeling isn't rational or try to downplay your emotions until they go away. People who have children, yes, even (and especially in my experience) men, will tell you what you should feel, think, or do the whole time you're pregnant, so take this time before you tell people you're pregnant to come up with ways to thank them for their concern but assure them you have your feelings and the safety of your baby well in hand. You don't need to drink the pregnancy Kool-Aid because a man, who has a wife, who was pregnant twenty years ago, told you to look happier because his wife said pregnancy is the best thing that ever happened to her. You can find a way you're comfortable with that shuts him down without allowing your hormones to take over and tell him to buzz off because he's never had a baby.

If your pregnancy is anything like mine and the moms I know, you're going to be exhausted during this phase of pregnancy. Let yourself rest; you'll get your energy back in the second trimester and will be able to accomplish more of what you think you need to. A downside of needing so much rest is your brain isn't always functioning at its peak. As a result, you can easily begin to forget things. Make a habit of writing things down or keeping notes in your phone so you don't have to remember it all by yourself.

I used to joke I wish I'd taken an IQ test before and during my pregnancy because I felt like my ability to recollect information was so much different than what I'd been used to for the first twenty-eight years of my life. But, of course, it's going to change. You have a million more things on your mind now, and chances are you pay much more attention to your diet and body than you have before because it feels like it matters more now.

Be comfortable with needing reminders on things and have grace with yourself on forgetting tasks/conversations. It doesn't make you dumb; it doesn't make you scatterbrained; it means you're taking your energy and focusing it into more important things than remembering when your next appointment is off the top of your head. Reminder alarms, online calendars, and notebooks are amazing things. You don't have to keep everything in your head, and you'll find more peace writing them down instead of second guessing what you think you remember.

Do research on pregnancy limitations so you don't fall victim to unnecessary oppression for things that have been disproven by peer-reviewed research. The rules have changed a good bit since our parents were pregnant with us, and the doctors don't actually give you any information on this. They just confirm or deny what you ask or, in some situations, give you a list of rules without any information as to why you need to follow them. *So* find some books that have been peer-reviewed or are based off peer-reviewed works and dive in!

It was a gloriously righteous moment when I had scientific facts ready to, politely, tell a man I work with he was incorrect when he saw me drinking a cup of coffee pregnant and told me that was on the no-fly list, like it was any of his business in the first place.

Consider managing expectations early. As bad as it sounds, I wish I lied to my entire family about my child's due date. Two weeks before I was due, I was inundated with texts asking if the baby was here yet or I was headed to the hospital. Why would I not tell you if that was happening? Do you really need to ask unnecessarily and add more stress? Consider what you want to tell people about your pregnancy with your spouse before you tell people you're pregnant because once the cat is out of the bag, everyone expects you to instantly know everything. A perfectly valid response is "I don't know. We'll let you know when we do" or "We haven't thought about it yet. We're just enjoying the process for now."

Now is also a good time to talk to your spouse about your thoughts on hospital visits and at-home visits post baby. This is so early in the pregnancy timeline because I'd do this before you tell your family you're pregnant. That way, when you tell your family you're expecting, if someone automatically assumes they'll be in the room for the birth of their grandchild/niece/nephew/etc., you and your spouse are on the exact same page and can either spread their joy by letting them know they'll be a part of the experience or allow yourself to be more comfortable and keep your boundaries by telling them that's not part of your vision for the birth of your child.

Keep in mind that it is great to have these conversations early but that as the time draws closer to your delivery, you may change your mind on some things, and that is perfectly fine! You should not have to put on a delivery show if you don't want to, and you should be able to have as much support as you need if you want additional people there. Make sure to check with your hospital on delivery room allowances before committing to allowing people to enter the birthing room. I was only allowed my spouse and a doula at my hospital.

Snacks by the bed are essential. Yes, you get hungry at night, but more importantly, you can wake up feeling nauseous because you're so hungry during your pregnancy. Eating a little something, taking nausea medicine, if you were prescribed it, and rolling over for fifteen more minutes make your day start a lot easier than if you just try to get up feeling sick already.

Are you keeping the gender a secret? Do you want it to be kept a secret from you and your spouse? Or do you want to know and not tell your family? Are you terrible at keeping secrets and know you won't be able to hold anything back? When are you planning on telling people you're pregnant? Do you want everyone to know right away or would you rather have some time to enjoy your family growing with just your husband? Have these conversations with your spouse and come to terms with one answer together.

If you decide to find out but keep it a secret from your family, you need to prepare yourself for someone figuring the sex out before you're ready. And if they handle it immaturely, how to shut them down. We had someone hear my husband say "he" one day, and for the rest of the pregnancy, we had to hear her gloat about how she thought she knew what it was because she overheard us talking, and it made us feel like shitty parents right from the start.

So decide what you want to do but find a way to accept your plans may not go as intended and work though that bundle of tight emotions at the beginning. Looking back, the person who found out about our son early wasn't trying to make us feel like shitty parents, but because we were so set on keeping things a secret, we got it in our heads this was the first time we'd not been able to do what we'd set forward to do in regard to our kid, and it didn't feel good. He wasn't even born yet, and we'd already felt like we failed, so take away the added stress and pressure and know that the best-laid plans don't always come to fruition, but that doesn't mean you love your child any less. It just means when you say he or she a million times a month at home, it becomes difficult to cut those pronouns out of your speech in public.

If you're currently working, think about what you and your spouse can afford to do and if you'd like to be a working parent. I can almost guarantee one of the first questions you'll get after "When are you due?" from everyone will be "Are you going to keep working?" It's not that you owe them an answer; it's that they keep *asking*, so you'll probably want a response ready just to shut them all up. This is a recommendation only for family and friends; you should feel absolutely no pressure to tell your work early what you'll be doing, especially if you have benefits you could lose.

Second Trimester

Thirteen Weeks through Twenty-Seven Weeks

We decided to tell our families we were expecting in the second trimester, and I thought it would be a fun and happy experience. Instead, it ended up being incredibly anxiety-inducing. My husband and I both grew up in very Catholic, no-sex-before-marriage families, so instead of being excited to tell our families I was pregnant, I was having panic attacks at the thought of admitting something to them that would let them know we'd had sex.

The line between "you're married, so it's encouraged" and "it's premarital, so go rot in hell, you heathen skank" didn't exactly disappear in the year and half we'd been married. Just having to admit to our parents that we were having a kid was close enough to screaming at them we're banging that I hated every single second of what should have been a wonderful experience.

There's a whole generation of people who feel this way, and it's a very difficult barrier to cross. I knew our parents would be ecstatic they were having grandkids, but I still felt like I was going into cardiac arrest every time we told them. If this is also an issue for you, discuss with your spouse who is going to be the one to make the announcement before you're on your way to the visit. Giving them a gift that makes it obvious you're pregnant can save you from having to find the words to tell them, if you feel like you won't be able to get them out.

Before you tell people you're pregnant, decide what your comfort level is with people touching your stomach during your pregnancy and make sure you and your spouse are enforcing this rule together. For some ungodly reason, women who have had babies think it's their God-given right to touch other pregnant bellies, *and it absolutely is not.* If you don't want people touching you, tell them, and if they try to touch you anyways, remove them or yourself from the situation.

I absolutely did not want my stomach to be touched during my pregnancy. It made me instantly mad and nauseous and ruined whatever I was doing. I moved out of the way of hands so many times during my pregnancy and even smacked someone's hand out of the way once.

Just because you're growing a baby doesn't mean you have to let people violate your personal boundaries and make you uncomfortable. Feel free to make this an announcement when you tell people you're pregnant. We didn't, and it led to a lot of repeating ourselves. If you want to be touched and share that experience with people, there are plenty of people who automatically go for it, but you'll also get really good at reading awkward pauses to know when people want to ask but don't know how to.

Find a good woman friend to discuss things with, preferably a mom who has done this before or someone who is also pregnant. My husband is an amazing person, but since he lacks a vagina and has never felt any of the aches and pains associated with a period or growing a child, sometimes, I felt more heard talking to someone who had been there before.

I was one of the first in our family and friend group to start having kids, so I didn't really have anyone to talk to who had been there before. There are resources online now to find moms in your area if that's what you want, but being a more private person, I preferred someone I had known for a while. So I chose a friend who was a two-time aunt and has a mom and mother-in-law who are doulas, so she's been exposed to pregnancy and birth a good bit for someone who hasn't yet had a kid of her own. Sometimes, it was a lot nicer to be able to vent to her so she could at least empathize that cramps suck and that they can make you want to lay down and groan on the bed for five minutes because your whole body is aching while it feels like your uterus is trying to cleave itself from the rest of your body.

People get so excited for the baby that besides asking "How are you feeling?" and then completely ignoring what you've said or adding a useless platitude, they can forget you're human too and only want to talk about the baby. People know you're pregnant and stop asking how work is going, if you've been keeping up with your hobbies, how is your mental strain since you're about to have your whole world be upended, you know, normal conversation stuff. It's disheartening how few conversations you get to have while you're pregnant that are about only you; so much of it always loops back to the baby after fifteen seconds of conversation, so feel free to set boundaries and to bring the conversation back to you at any time. Even just finishing a quick update about the baby and then jumping into "this is what I did at work this week" or "we have a vacation planned for (this) month" can help throw off people enough that they return to more normal topics.

Make sure talking about the baby isn't stressing you out. If you're having a difficult pregnancy and you'd like to not talk about the baby more than you've had to at appointments, make sure to let people know that. If you don't feel like telling your whole extended family, ask a parent or sibling to send out that text for you so you don't have to respond to follow-up texts.

During the last month of my pregnancy, if someone texted me asking about my baby or when it would finally be here, I'd ignore the text completely if they hadn't texted me in the last two months and taken the time to ask how I was doing personally or something as simple as sending me a meme, anything to show they cared at all besides just wanting baby updates.

There is a lot of research that goes into what to do for your health and for the baby's health and how to generate a list of items you'll need for the baby. It's a huge mental load for something that seems like it should be all fun but ends up feeling like a chore. It's really easy to think you need to do all these alone since the information about your health and the baby's directly impacts what you do and eat. Unfortunately, even if you release some of this control to your spouse, you can feel defensive or annoyed when they tell you what you can and cannot do with your body. Find a way to delegate here. This is the first real floodgate of additional things to do for the baby that can become overwhelming, especially since you probably know the sex by now and are also working through name selections at this time. If you feel like you can't delegate any of the research, have your spouse work on cleaning or cooking more often so you have time for research without becoming overloaded or staying up later since you're supposed to be getting lots of sleep.

The financial strain of having a baby can sit at the forefront of your mind and stress you and your spouse out if you feel like you're unsure what the future holds. Baby items are like wedding items; they're specifically marketed to a certain group of people and, as a result, are significantly more expensive. Don't get stuck in the mindset that you need to purchase all the things on online registries. Buy cheaper things like a dog bed instead of a "baby cushion" and be conscientious about what you need versus don't need. See appendix 3 at the end of the book for ideas on how to save money and manage the baby registry.

I'd recommend trying to live by what your new after-baby budget will be during your pregnancy and know that adding a child could add up to $400/month, after the big start-up stuff is purchased. That $400 does get cut in half if you can exclusively breastfeed; just remember, while that might be the plan, not everyone can breastfeed exclusively. If you're really struggling to live by a postbaby budget, consider where you can cut back or meet with a financial advisor to get your finances in order. Living by your postbaby budget a little earlier is a great way to build up some extra savings right before a very expensive time and, if you're thinking about not returning to work, to make sure you can afford to quit.

If you think something is wrong with your body and your OB keeps telling you "you're pregnant, just expect pain," make an appointment with your general care doctor. In my experience, they're much less likely to tell you it's just because you're pregnant and actually try to help you. Will you get pain just because you're pregnant and there are additional hormones and chemicals flowing through your body? Yes, you will, and I'm not saying blow everything out of proportion. I'm saying if you feel deep in your gut something is wrong, don't let someone write you off because you're pregnant, because they'll sure try to. I was getting tons of migraines during my pregnancy, and after being put off multiple times by my OB, I met with my PCP who quickly figured out I was drinking so much water every day that I was diluting the electrolytes in my body too much. All I had to do to stop my migraines was drink one electrolyte drink every day, which was an incredibly easy fix, but I wouldn't have known about it without going to my PCP.

There are a million things people/doctors/chiropractors/pelvic floor therapists/massage therapists/etc. are telling you to do to feel better. Do what you can to help with what hurts most, find ways to do things at home, and don't stress about the rest. You're going through *a lot,* so something has to give with the twenty-four hours you're given each day, and not every fix is going to be right for every person. Stretching is a big thing that can be done at home and doesn't require you to go somewhere to get some relief, so develop an excellent stretching routine and look into some stretches your partner can help you do to avoid multiple trips to the chiropractor/massage therapist.

In my experience, when you go into public where people can see you're pregnant, people, but men mostly, will congratulate you on being pregnant and then check that you're actually pregnant, like they didn't think to ask before they congratulated you or just keep their mouth shut if they're unsure. *So* having a response or easy exit strategy prepped besides annoyed glaring is a good idea. It's mostly fun to get congratulated, but when someone makes a huge deal of double-checking you're not just fat, the hormones can make you want to snap at them and then rant to your partner about it for the rest of the trip.

Telling your job you're pregnant and experiencing coworker's reactions are interesting experiences. It can come with the immediate question if you'll continue working, usually from younger employees who are just curious and not bosses (if you have good bosses), unsolicited advice, and, in some cases, the outright assumption you'll be leaving to stay at home. Some people then ignore the fact that you're pregnant and don't ask again, and others bring it up every time you're in a meeting with them. The first group is fun to share the experience with; the second group can make you self-conscious that you're taking up valuable meeting time week after week because they always remember new advice later and have to start with their weekly lesson.

For the repeat offenders, it's nice to have some work one-liners since these are relationships you need to preserve and not just strangers you'll never see again. Depending on your coworkers, they might have the best intentions or are going to be in your shoes soon, so you're happy to talk to them. When it's not someone with good intentions and they feel the need to bring up your pregnancy or imply you'll be gone soon, shut them down quickly and feel free to go to HR if you've addressed the issue and it continues to be a problem.

If you're going to make meals and freeze them before the baby comes and you're planning on doing a mass meal prep, instead of making a few extra servings every night for a few months, do it here and freeze it. Your body feels *amazing* now because your energy is higher than it has been in weeks. Take advantage of this time to do the things you need to prepare for the baby since it'll only get harder from here. I can promise pizza, Chinese food, and fast-food are not what your body wants after giving birth or right before giving birth when you're too tired to cook, so have something nutritious in the background waiting if you want it. If you want to meal prep but don't have any ideas what to cook, there are whole websites dedicated to baby arrival meal prep you can access online.

Holiday and birthday shop! It sounds silly, but you have the energy to do it now, and unless you're an exclusive online shopper, this is a great time to think ahead and get it done so you can hide everything in your closet and just pull it out when you need it. My baby was born in November, so I did all my Christmas shopping in June of that year, and wow, was it nice! No running out to get things for twelve people a month after my baby was born and sitting and wrapping it all. I could just roll up for Christmas with the bag I packed six months earlier, hand over the presents and my baby, and take a nap!

As soon as I started to feel my baby kick, I was instantly even more connected to him. I immediately wanted to settle on a name so I could stop calling him "baby" and talk to him using his name. It was unsettling to me how much my husband did not seem to feel this initial connection to our child until he could also feel the kicks, which took many more weeks and some good timing. What I wasn't understanding at the time was we both used the same indicator to feel that extra bond lock into place; however, it took my husband longer to feel it due to the logistics of babies. During the time in between when I was feeling the kicks and waiting for my husband to feel them, I felt like he didn't understand why I was pushing for a name and how close I felt to my baby, and I was worried he wasn't bonding to our child well. It was incredibly frustrating for me to feel like I was waiting and waiting and waiting for us to come up with a name when I was feeling this connection with a human I couldn't call by a name.

You feel these kicks and flutters and your life is completely altered again since at this point, you're already taking care of them via the food you eat, water you drink, vitamins you take, etc., but your spouse doesn't get those same instinctual signals, which can cause a gap in what you're feeling and when you're feeling it. Expressing your emotions to your spouse can be very hard at this time since putting your feelings into words can be difficult. Take some time to sit in your feelings and understand why you're feeling the way you are so you can better explain it to your spouse. Instead of telling your spouse you want something done because you just need it done, you can verbalize why this is so important to you and come to a (usually) much better resolution without stiff-arming your spouse or failing to get them motivated enough to work on something.

I get into the different tests you can expect to see during your pregnancy in appendix 1, so just know, for now, there is a test called the AFP, and it can be used to test for genetic abnormalities. I have a brother with open-back spina bifida, which can be genetic. This was always in the back of my mind during my pregnancy, and we knew it was a possibility before having kids, but we hadn't been overly worried about it. My results for my AFP for spina bifida came back almost thirty-five times higher than a usual singleton baby's results, and it absolutely shattered me. I was shaking and holding back tears when I hung up the phone and was sobbing the second I hit end. It was upsetting to think our baby would be less than healthy, but more heart shattering, all I kept saying in my head over and over was "This is my fault. I gave him the bad genes. He's going to have a less than perfect life because of me."

That kind of self-crimination is crushing! We got our AFP results at eighteen weeks, and the in-depth body scans are usually done at twenty weeks. So for two weeks, I completely despaired and would weep on and off at seemingly random times. My husband was so supportive and tried to convince me not to panic and that this was not my fault, but nothing stuck. I was too immediately in my head with recriminations to hear anything else.

Two weeks passed, and we went for the body scan of our baby, *and he was completely fine!* All this to say that diagnostic tests are great, and they can make sure you're seeing the right specialists, if there is a chance your pregnancy is more risky or there is something wrong with your baby. However, they are not always right, and you should do your best to remember that before spiraling and getting any real proof that something is truly wrong. You're going through more than enough already without adding that additional burden before knowing if there is actually something to worry about. Do your best to decrease the wait time between bad news and testing/scans that can confirm if there's anything to worry about, but besides that, there's nothing you can do, and you're just making yourself sit in those feelings of stress/worry/anger/depression more than you have to. Any time strong emotions begin to hit, sit down, close your eyes, and focus on breathing slowly and working through those emotions until they're resolved.

I have a family history of blood clotting conditions, and while I'm not positive for the gene, my OB thought it would be safest to take Lovenox, which is a daily subcutaneous (under the skin) injection that you put into your abdomen. I'm not a big needle fan. I used to be fine when I was younger, but now they give me the heebie-jeebies. However, every day, for seven months, I injected myself with Lovenox to take care of myself and my baby. It didn't matter that I had to stand in front of the mirror for five minutes some days and psych myself up, reminding myself that I was doing this for my baby, and I knew it wouldn't sting for very long afterward and that I am a powerhouse of a woman. It might have taken some time, but I still did it every day.

It's so easy to concentrate on the differences between your pre-pregnancy life and your pregnancy and feel like spending time focusing on new things you have to do that bother you makes you less of a mom. This. Is. Not. True. Take time to remember you are already a supermom, putting the health of you and your baby first by drinking water, getting sleep, eating, and stretching. Anything else you do in a day is just icing on the cake. Don't let yourself get down because you're apprehensive about doing something, wish you didn't have to do all these new things just to have a healthy baby, or want to stop doing something. You're still showing up every day and growing a human being, I mean, wow! What an awe-inspiring goddess you are!

Third Trimester

Twenty-Eight Weeks through Delivery

Remember the show *Kids Say the Darndest Things*? Well, there should 100 percent be a pregnancy version, and it would be funny but also not.

I had someone in a meeting tell everyone to stop complaining because I had to be the hottest person on the call (he clearly meant temperature). And what was I doing? I was sitting in my air-conditioned house on my computer, folding laundry, while my coworkers were on a construction site in an unair-conditioned warehouse in Brazil. I had someone tell me at my grandma's funeral that my mom was so excited in college to be a grandma one day. Now I know this isn't how she meant it, *but* am I just a means to a desirable end? Because that is what that sentence sounded like.

Certain people seem to panic and will word vomit things to you. If you have a repeat offender who continues to make you uncomfortable, find a time when the two of you (three, if you count the baby) are alone and address how they're making you feel. Let them know it's okay to not bring up the baby all the time and, if you want to, offer to keep them updated at a separate time, not in a group setting.

Perineum massages! A doctor never once said anything to me about these, but thankfully, we had a doula who pointed us in the right direction. If you're worried about tearing during a vaginal delivery, these can help you prepare your body to hopefully avoid or lessen tearing. You can google videos on how to do perineum massages, but you're essentially trying to teach your perineum, the area between your butt and vulva, to stretch and not be so tight. Get some gel or lube and practice these on yourself. I'd recommend starting before your belly gets too big because I started late, and my belly was big enough that reaching down there wasn't easy. So I had my husband do them instead of learning over time how to adapt to bending better. These can be awkward at first, especially if you have someone else help you with them, but they're a great thing to help your body slowly prepare for what's ahead, so they're worth the effort.

Stretch marks and how to avoid them. That's what everyone always talks about. Here's what they forget to talk about. Your skin can get so dry during pregnancy you feel like bugbites are covering your entire body. My belly and legs would get so dry I'd feel like fire ants were crawling all over me. Find a great lotion that will hydrate your skin but not leave a film of slime on your skin that will irritate you and make you want to wash the lotion off. It also helps to drink at least one gallon of water a day. Dry skin can be a sign of dehydration, so being hydrated should help reduce the amount of dry skin you see throughout your pregnancy.

I've always been a heftier person, so I love my snacks, but wow, have I never wanted to snack more than when I was pregnant. And not only did I want to snack, but sometimes, if I didn't snack, I would be so hungry I was nauseous and would have to lie down and shove crackers in my mouth like a hamster. By the end of my pregnancy, I had snacks in my office, bedroom, and basement for easy access. Make sure you find a way to have healthy snacks quickly accessible for when the hunger hits and turns into dizziness and nausea. I found prepping snacks on the weekends really helped. I cut up vegetables and cheeses and shelled nuts so I had them ready to go if hunger hit quickly. If you're dedicating your time to something else as well (e.g., work, another child, etc.), you can become incredibly distracted by what you're doing and forget to eat until your body reminds you that pushing off meals is no longer a viable option, and by then, you're already in the nausea danger zone. I had a dietician tell me great snacks usually include two food groups and are between 150–300 calories, so try to prep snacks that follow those guidelines.

Make your spouse pack a hospital bag for themselves but don't nag them. I don't know what it is about husbands that makes them assume they have all the time in the world before the baby is due. I have multiple friends who have had babies who told me it was a battle to get their husbands to pack hospital bags in a timely manner. I had the same problem as well and felt like I was nagging and nagging and nagging until I finally told myself if my husband wears the same underwear and clothes for three days, that's on him, and I can't let it stress me out. The time in the hospital goes so fast that if he never changed but washed his face, put on a hat, and reapplied deodorant, I probably wouldn't have even noticed he didn't change or shower.

Sleep was not easy for me when I was pregnant. I'd toss and turn to the point I felt like I was keeping me and my husband up all night. The bigger my belly got, the more I started feeling like I was stealing the covers, and then my mind would keep me up wondering if I was bothering my husband. After weeks of struggle, I decided to make our king-sized bed with two twin sheets, one for me and one for my husband, and add separate comforters on top of those so my constant rolling to get comfortable didn't make me feel like I was waking up my spouse or need to constantly check I wasn't pulling too much of the covers off him at night. I mean, marriage saving tip right here.

Do you know what you want your birth to look like? Have you found the birthing plan from the hospital and gone through the entire document to ensure you understand all the questions? This is a great time to go through those documents so at your next doctor appointments, you can ask questions about anything you don't understand or want to know the risks/benefits of. Even if you don't want a birthing plan because you don't want to set expectations that you don't meet on delivery day, understanding the questions lets you know what could potentially happen and what you might want to be ready for.

Sometimes, answers to the birth plan questions might come up toward the end of your doctor appointments; however, a lot of doctor's offices have rotating schedules at the hospital, so you see as many doctors as you can for your appointments, but you'll get the doctor who is onsite whenever your baby decides it is ready to come into this world, which means they tend to let the nurses at the hospital review your choices with you, and then the doctor is informed of those decisions and shows up right before they help you push.

Go through and talk about your birthing selections with your spouse, but know you can change anything the day of. If you and your spouse are split on a decision, remember, you might be a team, but this is *your body*, so the final decision is yours, and it's your job to talk your spouse through your decision until they're comfortable with it.

Even if you're not planning on having a C-section, take the time to ask your doctor to explain the process of an emergency C-section to you. As you'll see in appendix 2, one of the scariest things the moms I know went through during child birth was an emergency C-section. They hadn't thought about the possibility at all, and it was a lot to absorb emotionally, and from an information standpoint, in such a short period of time. Knowing what you might potentially need to experience can help you be a little calmer the day of should something unplanned happen during your delivery. It never hurts to have additional knowledge floating around in your head; it can hurt to find yourself unprepared for something so life-altering.

I know I've touched on it a few different ways, but it still blows my mind how much people ignore you as a human during pregnancy. People would look at my stomach instead of my face while having a full-blown conversation with me and not be able to look away from my baby bump or, I swear, even realize they were doing it.

With my friends, it was easy. A joking, "hey, my eyes are up here" does the trick every time, and the tension is immediately gone in the laughter. Family, coworkers, and strangers are a little harder. The worst part is my brain would always try to make concessions for people: "well, she's never had a baby, so she doesn't know what she's doing," "she adopted a baby, so she's never had this feeling," "she had kids fifty-five years ago and is just trying to remember a younger day and age," and "he's not trying to start a new HR ticket; he's just ignorant," and on and on and on it goes, making you feel guilty for trying to set boundaries.

I swear baby bellies are like a magnet, so if you're not okay with having eye contact completely ignored in a conversation, then you should find a way to address the topics quickly and kindly. I truly believe not a single person who did this to me meant to completely ignore me as a person, but once it happens, it happens every time if something isn't said. This may not be a big deal to some, but to others, it can be incredibly irritating, so if this bothers you, find a way to pull their attention back to your face.

Most insurance companies will let you order your breast pump early but will not release the order for delivery until a month before your baby's due date. The retailer taking the pump order can read you descriptions about the pumps, but they don't provide why one pump is better than another. Reach out to the retailer early to get a list of pumps so you can review the models yourself and know which pump you want. While it might be tempting, do not order a mobile pump. Mobile pumps are great for when your supply is in and you just need to get what's inside of you out, but if you need to do any kind of pumping to increase your breastmilk supply, mobile pumps are not helpful. Breast pumps are so expensive that I'd recommend getting a pump that will be able to do everything you might potentially need, just in case you need to increase your supply. My lactation consultant recommended Spectra or Medela pumps if you have no clue where to start.

Before your baby is born, you'll need to find a pediatric doctor's office for them to attend. Since babies usually have to go to the pediatrician the day after you're released from the hospital, you need to call the pediatrician before they're due and get put on a waiting list. They'll take your name instead of the baby's, so don't feel like you need to have it all figured out before you call. If you're planning on breastfeeding, when you're looking for a pediatric office, try to find one with a lactation consultant on staff. It makes life much easier if you have issues breastfeeding to be able to see the consultant while at the doctor's appointment instead of making a separate trip somewhere else.

The you part about coming home. What? You mean delivery isn't the end of it? Nope, not at all! I was so excited at the thought of bringing my baby home that I did the bare minimum of prep for my recovery at home and didn't do any research into how I'd need support when I got home. I had diapers, cooling pads, and nipple pads made and a cart I'd put together to sit at the side of my bed filled with books, medicines, tissues, and anything else I thought I'd need for the first few days, but that wasn't enough.

As a result, there were a lot of Amazon orders or husband convenience-store runs the first few days after we got home. My husband went and picked up ice pads, Dermoplast, and heat packs for my stitches and back. I ended up getting a tailbone donut cushion, an inflatable donut cushion, and my prescriptions as well. Prep the best you can but know you'll most likely need someone to do a run to the store. I'd recommend all of the above being at home and ready to go except for the tailbone items, those were more unique to my situation, and the prescription since you won't get those until you leave.

Bring your own clothes to the hospital; they're much more comfortable at a time you're already not feeling great. For delivery, I'd recommend buying two labor dresses; make sure they unbutton/unsnap all the way to the neck. Not all of them do, and it made it hard for my son and I to do skin to skin immediately after delivery. Why two dresses? If your water hasn't broken by the time you get yourself into the first dress, chances are you're going to need that second one or you'll be switching into a hospital gown. If you're someone who prefers wearing undies instead of letting things hang out, I'd recommend at least three to four pairs. Yes, this is for before your baby is born. There are lots of fluids that can be released down there, and if that's really going to be what makes you comfortable, then it's nice to be able to change them out whenever you want. See appendix 4 for my recommendations on a hospital bag.

Your brain is running and running and running with last minute things to do, so it can be very easy to get caught up in to-do lists and trying to do things to induce labor. Your baby is going to come when it is ready, so try to do what you can to induce labor, if you're past your due date, but don't allow yourself to be stressed trying to do it all. Try to slow down and enjoy these last mommy-and-baby bonding moments. They're very special, and it feels different once your baby is in your arms. Something about not seeing the baby or knowing what it'll look like but feeling such a deep love for him or her is different than looking into the face of a child in your arms. It's also a little less stress inducing having a baby inside you than when they're doing their ear-piercing cries, so these moments are full of calm love instead of overwhelmed love.

What does your water breaking feel like? This one is hard because everyone is different. Here are a few examples, though, and you can see appendix 2 for others.

I have a friend whose water broke slowly over three days, to the point she didn't even know her water broke, and the doctor over the phone didn't think it had either. My water broke very quickly with what felt like a strong contraction and a fast gush of water. A different friend of mine had a gush of water, but no contraction feeling, followed quickly by a second larger gush of water. There are many videos online that can help you determine if your water broke, so I won't go into that here, but know this is different for everyone and can even be different pregnancy to pregnancy.

If in doubt, call your doctor. I thought mine had broken in the shower at one point, so I called my doula and doctor. They weren't sure, and I wasn't sure if it broke, so we went in to get checked, and it hadn't broken, but better safe than sorry, and the triage nurse was really understanding. How on earth are you supposed to know if your water broke when you've never experienced it before and there are so many ways it can happen? Don't feel any shame in not knowing if your water broke.

We don't ever want to think about this happening to us, but starting at thirty-five weeks, you probably want to keep a spare outfit, towel, and a super pad in any car or purse you take with you when you go out. If your water breaks explosively in public, it'll be much nicer driving to the hospital or home in a dry set of clothes.

Missing your due date and having to wait to meet your baby can be very depressing. You've been anticipating the day you'll meet your baby for forty weeks now, and the day finally came, and your baby is still too cozy to come out. This can bring about negative thoughts about how your body isn't ready for this and spiral you into "this isn't what I had planned" cycles. You can be doing everything anyone has ever recommended to induce your labor, and your baby still might not be ready to meet you yet, and that can make you feel like a failure for something that isn't your fault.

Try to stay positive and remember your body is awesome, and you're just growing your baby a little more, which, until forty-two weeks, isn't bad at all! The good news is you know your baby will be there by 41.5 weeks at the latest, so you have a new day you can start counting down to. Try to find things to distract you during the day or after work, so you don't spend time ruminating on when you get to meet your baby. Relaxing nighttime routines really help your mental health and can convince your body you're not stressed, so your baby is safe to come out.

Missing your due date is even more frustrating when your family and friends are constantly badgering you, asking, "Have you gone to the hospital yet?" "Are you doing x, y, and z to induce labor?" "Isn't it weird that you and your husband were born a week early but your baby is over a week late?" blah, blah, blah. Keep your mental sanity boundaries in place, and if people are texting you repeatedly and it's bothering you, either ask them to stop or have someone like your mom or spouse mass text a group of family and friends to say they'll text everyone when the baby is on the way but to leave you alone for now. At the opposite extreme, if it helps you to talk about it, blow up every contact in your phone and vent to them about your frustrations.

So many women get wrapped up in the "this is what I said I was going to do" or "this wasn't my plan" that they stress themselves out. Don't feel bad changing your birth plan the month before, the week before, the day before, or thirty seconds before your child's birth (unless you suddenly want an epidural because it can be too late to change your mind on this if you wait until the last second). As a first-time mom, you didn't have any idea what to physically, mentally, or emotionally expect, so you're encouraged to listen to your body and adjust as necessary.in the moment. If your body ends up telling you to do something that wasn't in your original plan, then adjust your plan and feel good knowing your body and instincts have been preparing for this for almost ten months, so they'll see you through to the end.

If you're getting induced, ask if they need to do the IV right away. I did not know to ask this, so I had my IV done immediately and then had to have it sitting in my hand for over thirty hours; twenty-four of those hours, it wasn't even hooked up to anything. I had it placed, and I was put on an IV drip for the first hour, and then when I got it unhooked to go to the bathroom, the nurse said I didn't need it hooked up again. But I still had to pee in a hat (a plastic bowl in the toilet) since the IV had been started, and there was loads of pressure in my hand anytime I got up and had it down by my side. If I went to push my hair out of my face or redo my braid, my hair got caught in the tape or on the catheter. I had to have a glove placed on my hand and taped up when I went to take a shower the first night, and they didn't hook it up to anything again until I was getting ready to push almost twenty-four hours later. The nurse I had on my second shift seemed to think it was dumb that I already had an IV in, so if it seems like they're placing it early, I'd ask if they can wait a little longer before giving you the IV. It never hurts to be told no, and maybe you'll get to avoid some of the discomfort for a while.

The instructions I got at the hospital for pushing were *terrible*! I really wish I was joking when I say they told me to "just push how it feels right" when I had an epidural and couldn't feel anything. So my recommendation for pushing: I'd advise starting with pushing from the abdomen down, and then if that doesn't work, change it up. After I'd pushed for four hours, the doctor came in and told me to push from the abdomen down, and we progressed *so much* faster after that. Besides that...pushing, what's it like?

When I was ready to push, the nurses put my legs into stirrups (since I couldn't move them myself) and told me to give one ten-second push. A contraction hits, and you take a deep breath and then sit up and push for ten consecutive seconds, the nurses count for you. Then you lay back and take a second to breathe and do it again two more times. You repeat the whole process at the next contraction. I would *heavily* recommend breathing practices at home to prep for this. Since I didn't do breathing exercises during my pregnancy and my lungs were being compressed by the baby, a count of ten was already hard without pushing. The deeper the breath, the more pressure to help push the baby out, so make sure you're practicing deep breaths and letting them out as soon as they're as deep as you can go. Don't hold your breath while practicing unless you talk to your doctor first, and they're okay with it.

Hospital Time

Active Delivery through Hospital Release

Your delivery and recovery time at the hospital are so short, compared to your first forty weeks, and your life is changing so drastically you don't really have time to absorb your feelings too much at the hospital. As a result, this is a relatively short section. Appendix 2 will give you some insight into what your time at the hospital can look like, but here are some emotional things you might need to deal with during this time:

I thought I might be mildly traumatized by being forced to have strangers looking deep into the soul of my vagina while I pooped on a table, but I could not have cared less. There is *so much* going on when you start to push, there is an entire team of professionals walking you through the process, you're thinking about what you need to do next, what your baby is going to look like, so the time went by really fast and I didn't even think to be embarrassed...even when I could tell I was pooping on the table. Even though the nurse was as discreet as she could possibly be, I still knew. Delivery nurses are awesome and clean shit every day they are working. I can promise you they've seen so many other women poop before that your poop does not faze them, so don't let it faze you.

Delivery was hard for me. I go into the details in appendix 2, but long story short, because of my pain afterward, my husband held our son for the first two-ish hours of his life, and I sat puking and fluctuating between cursing up a storm and feeling miserable. I had an intense bond with my son before he was born and felt my husband was hardly bonded to him, but as soon as my son was born, I felt like we did a complete 180, and my husband was the one who had this strong bond with our son, and I felt like he wasn't even mine even though I had almost thirty hours of labor to prove he was. My whole life, I had wanted to be a mom; and the second I had accomplished what I wanted, it was like I had been given a random child to look after.

What I didn't know at the time was after I recovered from the pain and got through the "oh, shit, what do I need to do now" phase, my postpartum depression (PPD) kicked in, and I didn't feel like I really bonded to my son until I stopped breastfeeding, and my PPD went away. Did I love him with all my heart? Absolutely! Would I do anything to ensure he was taken care of and safe? You bet your ass! Did I feel like this tiny little human in my charge was a part of me? No, I did not for the first six and a half months of his life. Your body and mind need time to process and adjust to everything you just went through. If you don't feel bonded to your baby right away, that's okay; it will come with time. You'll make it through this and be better than you imagined you could be.

After delivery, we spent enough time in the delivery room to get my pain under control before we moved to the recovery suite. Immediately, they helped me breastfeed my son. Again, there should be absolutely no embarrassment here for any of this! In any other circumstance, would five people watching you whip your boob out for the entire world to see be weird? Yes. But this is their job; they're not interested in your mom titties. No offense, I'm sure they're lovely.

Once you learn how to breastfeed, you've learned how to make your baby stop screaming and be comfortable, which is an amazing magic trick. These babies are going from having constantly full bellies and being warm and cozy to a cold hospital room and learning what hunger is. Babies can be pretty upset for the first few hours of their lives, trying to adjust to these new sensations, so learning how to sooth them quickly will save you and your spouse lots of headaches.

Be prepared to get some cramps during breastfeeding. Your uterus is already trying to shrink, so that doesn't help, but just know breastfeeding, throughout the life cycle of your breastfeeding journey, can cause cramps at any time. The nurses have access to hot packs and cold packs, if you feel like you're cramping, and one of those would help. Ask them if you can have some of those to alleviate the pain. You're already taking pain medicine to try and mitigate the pain, but it won't get all of it, I promise, so the hot/cold packs can help. The nurse on my second day explained that they try to keep your pain below a five without overmedicating you, so based off the pain levels you give them when they come in and ask how you're feeling is how they medicate you.

I didn't have a complicated delivery with anything quickly worrying that popped up, so even when I was told we needed to use forceps, I didn't feel any panic since I'd had an hour of pushing to consider my options and become comfortable with my choice. I did, however, feel panic when I had to confess to the recovery nurse that even though I felt like my bladder was going to explode, I suddenly forget how to pee even though I'd been successfully controlling that for the past twenty-five years of my life. Be patient if you need some time to figure out how to pee again. They had me stand and sit multiple times and try squatting versus sitting and several other things before I could find the muscle again that let me pee. They know to expect lingering loss of control, and they know how to walk you through it. They are not going to let your bladder explode. They can catheterize you if they need to even though this is far less comfortable without an epidural since you'll feel everything. Take deep breaths to help relax your mind and body. Relaxing can loosen your bladder muscles, and the deep breath can put added pressure on your bladder. The more relaxed you can get, the easier this process will go.

The second time I panicked after delivery was when the lactation consultant had gone home for the day, and I felt like I couldn't get my baby to latch onto anything but the finger I was shoving in his mouth. I tried self-expressing and couldn't get anything out, and no one was there to help me. We called the nurse in, and she brought in a pump for us to use to try and get some colostrum out that we could then use a glove to get into the baby's mouth. The nurses might not be certified lactation consultants, but they've been around the block a time or two and can be very helpful to first-time breastfeeders. Just because the lactation consultants have gone home for the day doesn't mean you don't still have help, and even if you're a severe case and your nurse has tried absolutely everything and nothing is working, the hospitals keep formula (and sometimes donated breastmilk) on hand that could hold you over until the lactation consultant can get to you. They're not going to let your baby starve, and it's normal for babies to lose weight before they go home. They're going from a constantly plugged in supply of food to needing to learn how to notify you they're hungry and how to eat. It's a steep learning curve, so there's some wiggle room built in there.

I mentioned hot packs and cold packs for breastfeeding cramps before, but know you can use these for any nonbaby-related muscles as well. Pushing for multiple hours can make things like your biceps, abs, and lower back sore, so having those packs can help you get over some of the original soreness more quickly. Also ask your spouse for help getting up and moving! I was so convinced I needed to get back into moving right away that I ignored all my incredibly sore muscles and would just pull myself up to go to the bathroom, forgetting that I'd been using those same muscles to push during delivery for five hours, so they were already *way* past their normal tolerance for working out. I should have been having my husband push my body into a sitting position or using the automatic bed to sit up instead of tiring those muscles out even more when they were already past their max use point. This is really important to do at the hospital because if you're consistent about using help at the hospital, by the time you get home to your bed, your muscles have recovered enough that they can begin working again without too much soreness, and you can do simple things like get up to pee without too much, if any, help.

Do not let the nurses make you feel like shit for sending your baby to the nursery. *Do not let the nurses make you feel like shit*

for sending your baby to the nursery. Do. Not. Let. The. Nurses. Make. You. Feel. Like. Shit. For. Sending. Your. Baby. To. The. Nursery! Go show this book to your spouse and have them read that last line to you just so you can really hear it and feel it in your soul.

The first nurse we had was very kind and knew I was coming off the pain medicine hard, so when we couldn't get our newborn to stop crying after breastfeeding him, she offered to take him to the nursery so we could get a few hours of sleep before I had to feed him again. I wasn't sure how to feel about letting him out of our sight at first, but utter exhaustion and the overwhelming need to cry won out, and we let her take him for a few hours. And, wow, do you need that. Remember, you've been up for God knows how many hours at this point have just gone through bodily trauma, and to be a patient and kind parent, *you need your sleep.* Sleeping for even a little bit makes a world of a difference in how your body reacts to your baby crying. Sleep keeps you from going into the sheer panic of "Why won't you shut up?! All these new moms are going to think I'm a bad parent, and I can hear when their baby is crying, so I know they hear you" instead of just thinking about how uncomfortable your baby must be and giving them the comfort and help (warmer clothes, food, being burped, etc.) they need. Some nurses will not offer to take your baby to the nursery, so if you feel like you really need a break, you need to ask them to take your baby to the nursery for a little and then… *do not let the nurse make you feel like shit for sending your baby to the nursery.*

Master trick: if your baby is already crying and you want the more refusal-inclined nurses to cave and offer to take them to the nursery, go hold the baby by the door of your bedroom suite instead of deep in the room. The nurses can hear the baby louder if you stand by the door and, in my experience, are more likely to come and see if you need a break, if not only for your sake but also for the other moms around you so they can get some rest too.

If you hurt your tailbone during delivery, immediately order a donut online while in the hospital or stop on the way home at a pharmacy to get one. The longer you wait, the more pain will build up. If it's been a few weeks and there's no improvement, call your doctor to see if you can have a checkup before your six-week appointment and ask if you can go to physical therapy. I hurt my tailbone and hadn't even realized it in the hospital because of the initial recovery pain, soreness, and superior drugs; however, I was positive by two weeks that something was definitely wrong with my tailbone, so I called and went in early. If some things feel like they're recovering and others don't, at the very least, give your doctor a call and see if it's something they're concerned enough about that you should go in for a consultation.

You learn to adjust to sleeping differently while you're pregnant and think, *Ah, yes, I'm having this baby today. At least, I'll sleep well tonight.* Well, that thought may not be true and not just because you now have a baby to take care of. Sleep comfort is like the forty-week pregnancy myth; it's not actually forty weeks, and you need to expect to slowly go back to a new normal. Can you sleep on your back right away? Sure, but if you still have too much weight in your stomach area, your blood vessels might get a little squished and cause things to fall asleep while you sleep. Sleeping on my stomach was not an option for me. My boobs hurt so badly from nipple soreness that putting enough pressure on them to roll over was a no-go. And my hips still hurt when I would sleep on them due to the added weight pushing down on them. Expect to still be rolling around for a few weeks at the very least, especially those first two nights in the hospital bed, oof.

Fourth Trimester

Returning Home through Finding Your New Normal

Before we get into anything else and before you even go to the hospital to have your baby, try to arrange to have a support team close by to help you in the days after you return home. My husband and I made a "rule" with our families that we wanted two weeks to adjust as a family before we had anyone come to our house, and we made it three days before we called my parents over to nap and recoup.

You're not unfit to be a parent, and you're not failing. You're exhausted, and your body is recovering from trauma. If you got much sleep in the hospital postpartum, you are a lucky duck since nurses are in at all hours of the night to poke and prod you and the baby, and when they're not there is miraculously when the baby needs to try to figure out what the heck it does with a nipple to get food. Phone a friend and take a nap! It'll make you a more patient parent, and you'll enjoy those first days with your baby more instead of being overwhelmed.

Originally, we didn't want anyone at our house so we could get comfortable as a family, and I wouldn't have to worry about feeling like I was confined to the floor our room was on when company was over. Then we had our baby and hardly slept the entire time we were at the hospital. So by the time we got home, we were absolutely exhausted and needed a break. We asked my parents to come over and watch the baby, and, *wow,* was that way better than struggling through life for two weeks to meet our initial expectations. Your entire world is changing rapidly, and you're doing the best you can to forecast and plan for the future, but sometimes, the future isn't like you think it'll be, and knowing when to ask for help is critical during new parenthood.

Do not expect to have "normal" sleeping and waking hours during the first few weeks, if not months, of your baby being home, and do not feel pressure to respond to people during "normal hours" either. You are being constantly overstimulated, learning new things, and adapting to a new way of life, all while sleep deprived. Your friends and family can wait to get a response. We're so addicted to our phones nowadays that we try to constantly be responding to texts/calls or updating social media, and that's not realistic with a new baby. Even if you have time to respond, sometimes, instead of responding, you need to let your brain not think about anything and watch feed videos or a rerun TV series. Allow yourself grace in response times, and if someone doesn't understand your need for more time, tell them point-blank you'll be late in responding. And if they still don't seem to get it, invite them to your house to wash bottles and pump parts, do laundry, make dinners, do dishes, buy diapers, etc., all while you peacefully hold your baby, and when they leave exhausted, they'll get it.

In these early days, it's very easy to hide if you're not doing well. A simple "I'm tired" or "my body hurts" is so easy to pass off, and while that is also true, it's not always the true reason you're feeling off. It's hard to admit you need help or you're not doing well mentally and have the strength to ask someone to step in, but it can put you in a much better and safer place.

We talked about getting to a great place of openness with your spouse in the zeroth trimester, and this will really test it. It's very hard to look into the eyes of someone you love, who you want to love and respect you, and tell them something as serious as you've been thinking about killing yourself or hurting your baby. The NIH says between 6.5 and 20 percent of women experience PPD; that's not an insignificant amount. If you're having thoughts of self-harm or of harming your baby, you *need* to let somebody know. PPD and PPA (postpartum anxiety) are very serious conditions that can be lessened with the aid of medicines and/or therapy. Protecting your baby from worldly threats is your job, so taking them out of a situation where you could potentially hurt them means you're being a *great mom*. Your body will recover from this, you will recover from this, and your baby will get to live to an age where you get to see them without this fog of mental illness around you, and that will be a beautiful day. But you have to hold on until that day by getting the help you need and deserve.

If you choose to breastfeed, you will get mad at your spouse for having useless nipples at some point in time, which sounds funny now, but when they hand you the baby after only having it for fifteen minutes and say, "I think they're hungry," you'll just want to titty twist their useless nipples until they come off and you can throw them on the ground and stomp on them. Or when they're snoring while you breastfeed your baby, you'll be sitting there, fuming, and then you can finally go to bed because the baby is done eating, but you're still so mad that their nipples are useless that you can't sleep during this short, glorious window when you actually could be sleeping. It doesn't matter if they got up and changed the baby before they handed it off to you; you're still doing most of the feeding and getting the least sleep at night.

Breastfeeding is for champions, and milk coming in takes time. You might feel alone in this part of baby care, but remember, it also frustrates your spouse to see you going through things they cannot step in and help with, so getting mad at them isn't going to help the situation. Find ways that they can support you and take pressure off in other places so when you get mad at their useless nipples, you can remember they're doing X so you don't have to. There is nothing like being woken up by a screaming infant with no warning, getting your nipples yanked on to feed them at ungodly hours of the night, and being smacked in the face, headbutted (feeding frenzy), scratched, and throat-punched, all while your husband sleeps soundly, so find a balance so you can find the peace.

I think there's a widely spread misconception that when you have your baby, you recover from whatever happened during delivery (vaginal stitches/stretching or C-section incision), and you're able to move on to the next stage of parenting. I found this to be wildly untrue. I took too much comfort in the fact that women have been having children for centuries, and my body would be able to recover and move on without too much additional effort from me.

Every journey is different, but after my son was born, I was attending physical therapy, seeing a chiropractor, and seeing a massage therapist. Although I'm really not begrudging that last one. There's really nothing better than handing your baby off to your husband to go get a medically recommended massage. I also had an X-ray, abdominal ultrasound, colonoscopy, steroid injection, and emergency room visit, all within seven months of having my baby. This was on top of all the effort I had to put into breastfeeding since my production was not nearly enough to support my son (and never fully got there, *this is okay,* and we'll talk about it later) and the struggle to regain intimacy with my husband between both of us being exhausted from our new life pace and from sex being physically painful the first few times. So please take the time to mentally prepare yourself for these possibilities and know they are going to potentially take time out of your already swamped schedule, but it's important for you to make time to mentally and physically recover from everything you went through.

You're going to get over this stage, but since no one was honest with me, I'll be honest with you. You're going to have a rough next couple of months. I'm not trying to scare you. I'm trying to let you know that you should be gathering your support system to help you through this time, let you heal, and let you sleep. You and your spouse do not need to be in this alone. Even if you don't have friends and family willing to help, there are doulas that provide post-birth services and can help you get your feet under you if need be.

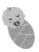

If you had a vaginal birth, when you get home, make sure you're taking the sitz baths that the doctor recommends. Even if you don't think they're doing you much good, it's a medically recommended reason to get twenty to thirty minutes to yourself, and you *need* that. It gives you time to let your body come out of panic mode and allows your brain to start settling as well. It also can help reduce the itchiness for your stitches. If you want your stitches to heal more quickly, make sure to sit under a fan and let those stitches dry out for a bit before getting dressed again.

I was shoveling down calories at the hospital, and then a few days after I got home, I realized I did not feel like eating or drinking at all for weeks after birth, but this is really important for milk production and for your body to heal, so snack and drink as much as you can so you can recover quickly and get that milk in.

Milk production is not always easy, and some moms need to spend lots of time pumping after feeding their baby so they can get their production levels up. Don't just expect your boobs to go from zero to 100 percent after your baby is born or even in a couple days. They need to adjust to your baby's needs. Sometimes, you can have too much milk already, and your baby can choke when they start feeding. Sometimes, there's not enough, and you have to supplement with formula. It's all a frustrating balancing game that you and your baby need to figure out so you can both get what you need from those interactions. If you have too much and donate it, excellent! If you have too little and have to supplement with formula, still excellent! You're putting the health of your baby above the societal pressure to only breastfeed, and that can feel disappointing some days, but you have to remember it's better for your baby to get the food they need than to go hungry and continue to lose weight because you're trying to demand more from your body than it can handle.

Your first poop. It's not fun, but you don't need to be as scared as I was. Start taking stool softeners immediately after birth. I had a colonoscopy done after my son was born, and the doctor said there was nothing about long-term MiraLAX use that would make your body less efficient in the future, so don't be afraid to take it as soon as you get home. There were lots of pressure and pulling on stitches, so you want your stool as soft as possible. Don't try to push it out, just wait until you really have to go, and let nature take its course. Squatty potties or yoga blocks can really help get your body into the correct position for pooping to make it easier on you. Just place them under your feet and relax the best you can on the toilet. I had something nearby that I could grab onto when the pressure got intense so I wouldn't try to clamp up my butt and make it harder to get the poop out.

Your first few nights at the house are full of insane mood swings. You'll hear baby sucking in the middle of the night, and you wake up instantly frustrated because you can't sleep, but they need to be fed, so you go to feed them, and your baby laughs while you're rocking them back to sleep, and it's so adorable you don't mind they woke you up after only thirty minutes of sleep. Then they have a nightmare and cry with their little eyes shut, just lying there, and your heart breaks a little, and you want to hold and sooth them. Then they gag or suck in air like they haven't been breathing for the last thirty seconds, and you fly out of bed in an utter panic to ensure you don't need to intervene. You end up feeling more emotions in the middle of the night than you used to in a whole day, and not only is being up to take care of the baby exhausting but the emotional strain all those fluctuations take on you is also draining. So like we've said before, do your best to have a support team that can help you make up some sleep during the day in those first few weeks after the baby is born.

For your sanity, find a way to turn a complaint into a positive thing each day. For example:

- ❖ There are so many dishes on the counter. → I was able to feed my family today.
- ❖ The laundry is piled higher than the basket. → We've been given/bought enough clothing we can get through the week without doing laundry.

❖ My spouse is "insert vice here" (e.g., golfing, videogaming, poker, reading, etc.) instead of helping me with the baby. → I have a spouse/partner who knows how to recharge to be the best parent they can be. I should take a page from their book.

❖ I'm exhausted all the time. → Being stuck in constant survival mode has taught me what and who is important in my life and has allowed me to more easily

- speak out when I don't like or want something or need help,
- respond to texts and phone calls when I feel ready instead of making them a priority,
- help filter down my hobbies to what really matters to me, and
- declutter my life. If I wear something or see something I hardly use, I'm much more likely to throw it out or put it in a Goodwill pile because I don't have time to sort through the stuff I don't like or want multiple times a week now.

It's easy to have lofty ideas before you have your kids of what you're going to feed them, how your future career will look, and how your interactions with your child and your spouse will be. It's *a lot harder* to remember what your goals and ideas were on how you want to parent when you've been awakened for the fifth time that night to feed a newborn who will not stop crying. Show yourself grace. You can change your goals and expectations on what having a child looks like now that you physically have a child to take care of and know what it's like. You can also put those goals on hold for the first few months until you can get to a place where you have the ability to work on those. You're so sleep-deprived and constantly being pulled in a million different directions at first that it's hard to be a human, let alone practice gentle parenting 100 percent of the time.

My husband is the most patient person I have ever met in my life. I have given him *tons* of reasons to lose it on me over the years, and he's never once done it. Within a few days of having our son at home, my husband was frustratedly yelling at him to stop crying. There is nothing you can do to prepare yourself for the new life situation you're about to find yourself in, so tag team whenever possible so you can remain the person you want to be. Being awakened to feed a baby after forty minutes of sleep when you've only slept for eight hours in the past two days can make even the most patient of people short-tempered. Your kid is not going to remember if you yelled at them to stop crying or gave them store-bought baby purees. Do what you need to do to navigate this phase of your life in a way that protects you, your spouse, your child, your marriage, and your family. Everything else can fall by the wayside for a while if it needs to.

Remember to tell your spouse you love them. We can get caught up in running up to the baby and expressing our love for them, but you need to remember your spouse/partner was your first love, and if you want your baby to have a healthy sense of relationships, they need to see the two of you model one. If your spouse is coming into the room and snuggling the baby and then going to leave a gentle reminder that mommy needs snuggles too is always a good way to make sure you're getting the comforting love you need as well.

Moms and dads have very different mentalities on how to get through the day. I told my husband I had started microdosing pre-workout to have enough energy to get through the day, after I'd stopped breastfeeding, and then had to listen to him tell me I shouldn't be doing that and endure his judging stare when he saw pre-workout on the counter in a cup. I told other moms I knew I'd been doing that, and the nurse and doctor at my general care office, who were also moms, and all of them said you do what you have to do to get through the day sometimes. The spouse who isn't in the trenches every day isn't going to see how much you're struggling to find the energy to do things when they're not around and, as a result, doesn't tend to understand why you do what you do and downplays the situation or gives you solutions that don't work (i.e., taking a nap in the middle of the day). Kids are notorious for behaving differently parent to parent, so your spouse might not understand what all needs to do done in a day or how draining your kid(s) can be for you. Do what you gotta do on the hard days, momma; it won't last forever.

There is nothing as amazing as watching your family fall in love with your child, more specifically seeing the love grow between your spouse and you child, but there's also a magic to watching your parents become grandparents and your siblings become aunts and uncles. You just added an extra member into the family, but this time, it wasn't like your spouse where they had a while to get to know them first and love them. This is a brand-new life that they're instantly and overwhelmingly in love with, and it's amazing to watch. On the other side of the coin, there are some family members who show no effort or desire to meet your baby, and that can be very hurtful, especially if it's someone you care about. It's hard, but making the effort to talk to them about it is very important if you want to preserve a relationship with that person. They might be so wrapped up in their own life that they don't understand how hurtful they're being. I've found people with no desire to have kids of their own one day are either instantly in love with your child, like it is their own, or they want to ignore the baby at first because this little intruder isn't a member of your group. Take things slowly and let them get used to the thought of a baby in their lives. It's a lot to adjust to.

While you have definitely front-loaded a lot, if not most or all, of the work of having a child and your body is taking a beating, please remember your spouse is allowed to have bad days as well. This is a new situation for the both of you, and when they complain about how exhausted they are, your brain might automatically default to something like this (best read as a rushed slew of words bordering on pissed hysteria):

> Really?! Because I don't remember you getting up with the baby five times last night or your nipples being sucked on until they're bruised and bleeding or you doing anything besides your normal nine-to-five and then watching TV while holding the baby, which was sleeping! At which point, I ran around the house and did the laundry, cooked dinner, did the dishes, cleaned all the bottles and pumps, and a million other things that needed to be done after having spent the day changing, feeding, burping, and educating our child while trying to squeeze in research about what they'll need to eat in the next six months and what brand of diapers is best for preventing blowouts—all while leaking blood out of a uterus that is cramping like a mother fucker as it attempts to shrink back to its normal size, but, yes, please let me hear how sitting on your ass at your computer all day is sooo taxing.

Instead of going into a rant that will surely start a fight or make your spouse feel like their emotions aren't valid, please take a breath and stop and listen to what they have to say. Yes, you need to listen to them and not just tune them out without saying any of the million things you want to yell at them about how you're worse off. They need to know they're being heard and their emotions are being understood. They're coming to you because they're feeling stressed and exhausted, and the worst thing you can do is push them away by telling them to suck it up or not being able to respond with compassion since you weren't actually listening to what they said.

This is not a competition. This is a life-altering experience that pushes you and your spouse to the brink and expects you to make it through to the other side as a unit so your child can still rely on two happy parents in the same household, which is asking a lot of a marriage. There were times my head just wanted to blow up with anger at my husband after our son was born, but those times were all when I was overly exhausted, needed a break, and felt like I was out of control because I was not getting anything done that I thought needed to be done in a day. Somehow, by the grace of God, I managed to hold my tongue every time I wanted to yell something like the above at my husband, and I'm very proud of myself for that because I know if I hadn't, I'd have felt worse in the end for saying all those things to him when we were both trying our best.

My six-week appointment was *very* disappointing. It's a physical checkup and a check-in to ensure I had a plan for contraceptives. Nothing else. And even though they told us multiple times at the hospital not to have sex before six weeks, one of the first questions I was asked was, "How does it feel when you have sex now?" Are you kidding me? You just told me not to do that. *Why* would you assume I had? They just made sure I had a plan in place for contraceptives and basically told me to leave and have a good life. They did not care if I couldn't squat down to pick up my baby without my tailbone throbbing and my incontinence flaring up.

There was no concern for my chafed nipples, and there was a lot of "yep, that's how it's going to be for a while" when I brought up my concerns about any pain I had. They were so unhelpful and unapproachable that I didn't even feel like my appointment was a safe place to discuss my PPD and was on the verge of frustrated tears the entire time. If you want helpful advice on how to best make it through this next few months of your life, use this book or find a mom friend who is a little farther ahead of their pregnancy than you are, but do not rely on your six-week appointment to be the help you need. Bouncing things off other moms helps tremendously and lets you validate your feelings by knowing you're not alone in what you're feeling (e.g., stress about baby breathing, how your baby is different with your spouse, extra mental weight the mom's carry, trying to find a new normal, how to fix cracked nipples, how to balance work/life/baby/marriage/household chores, conversations to have with your spouse before they stress you out too much, how to balance the workload, etc.).

I think OBs have become so desensitized by the number of pregnant and postpartum women they see every day that they've forgotten how completely overwhelming the entire process of pregnancy is. Not only do women have valid concerns about their body that they need helpful answers to but they also have hormones running through them the whole time that make their concerns even more frantic in their heads, and our society has no avenue to help these women. We just tell them to go home and leave them hanging to figure it out themselves. So instead of having one place we can go to repair our body and minds, we end up seeking out specialists on our own in the hopes we can somehow find some help, and those are only the lucky women. Some women don't have insurance that allows them to do that, so, instead, they go through this without the help of other medical providers. Don't let your OB push you out the door without help and don't be afraid to continuously circle back to your point if they give you nonanswers. Eventually, something helpful will come out.

I hope all your doctors have told you this, but just in case, having no period for months after delivery is possible if you're a breast-feeding mom, but *you can still get pregnant*, hence the sole focus on contraceptives at your six-week appointment. As long as you know this, I trust your absolute and utter exhaustion to keep it very clear in your mind that some form of birth control might be a good idea but as long as you know you can make your own decisions.

A sad thing about having a newborn is the ugly parts of the people in your life become more apparent. Instead of seeing people as unique and bringing a fresh perspective to things, your brain instead thinks, *I don't want my child raised like that*, and you try to shelter them from learning the "ugly" parts of the people in their lives and picking up those habits. This can make it very hard to leave them alone with people you don't fully align with and can make it hard to align with your husband on who the guardians of your children should be in the event of your untimely demise. This fades once you've had some time to let your child interact with the people in your life whom they'll call family, but it can make things seem more negative for a while and can have you feeling like an overly protective momma bear. There's nothing wrong with wanting to protect your children and save them from being raised a certain way, but don't swing the other way completely and have them grow up thinking the people they love aren't good enough.

"Breastfeeding mom's lose weight. It's a great way to get rid of the baby fat." Absolutely false in my experience. I could not lose a single pound while breastfeeding, and a month after I stopped, I was shedding weight with workouts and calorie management. My postpartum depression (PPD) also went away, and my areolas turned their normal color again instead of being darker than I'd ever tanned any part of my body to in my entire life, and I spent years as an outdoor lifeguard in Florida. The point is your body recovers after delivery, but you also go through another recovery after you stop breastfeeding when your hormones go back to a more "normal" level. So until you've stopped breastfeeding, know you could be doing everything in your power to lose weight or control your mental health, and it might not happen yet. Be patient and know the end is in sight.

It was cute when you were pregnant to go out to a restaurant, be sat at a booth, and have to push the table more toward your spouse to accommodate for your baby bump. It doesn't feel cute when you're seven months postpartum and sitting in a booth, thinking, *Dang, I wish I could push this back toward my husband without feeling like a whale.*

Baby fat can fall off or it can take some hard-earned work that your body might not be able to do during early recovery. I was not cleared by my physical therapists to do things like squats, jumping, running, etc. until ten months after my son was born, and even then, it was a "hey, build these skills up, know your body has to adjust, and your urinary incontinence will probably come back each time you start a harder workout until those muscles are strong again." It was one hell of a process, and I hated feeling like it was two steps forward and one step back, so if the weight isn't falling off like you'd like it to, know there are *so many* factors going into how your body is adjusting to get back to normal that you might have to be more patient with yourself. Nobody likes feeling bad about themselves, and it's worth remembering your body brought a life into this world and rearranged the majority of your internal organs to do it. Healing takes time, and the meaner you are to yourself about your slow progress, the more likely you are to take even longer to get to the you you'd like to see in the mirror again.

Bounce back mentality. Say it with me: *Fuck. That!* Your body just went through almost ten months of rearranging its organs to grow a human you then had to get outside of your body. You need time to let your organs rearrange themselves again, and you need time to readjust to your new lifestyle before you can worry about things like getting into your old pants.

I love that some women are physically and mentally able to work out soon after birth and feel confident enough that they post photos and videos online, but these women are not the norm, and you shouldn't let them be the norm in your mind. Working out too quickly can be bad for your body. I know a woman whose stitches started to come out just because she did too many stairs in her three-story house doing laundry and making meals for herself while recovering from childbirth. Make sure your doctor has approved you to return to working out if you're really antsy to get going again; otherwise, your recovery time may end up being longer than the originally estimated time.

Having a baby that is underweight can end up giving that baby more serious health conditions throughout their lives than if they're overweight, so I was happy to gain extra weight during my pregnancy and know I wasn't going to be potentially harming my baby by making sure I only ate exactly what I could, and as a result, I have some work to do to "get back to normal" and that's okay.

Allow yourself some grace and buy pants larger than your original prepregnancy pants and rock those. Your body is an amazing fortress and should be treated that way, not hated for taking time to return to your prebaby "normal." I had tons of stretch marks during my pregnancy that are still on my skin. I will never have a body that looks prepregnancy again from those alone, but I like to think of them as tattoos with a story now.

A midwife in my doctor's office told me it took nine months to grow that baby, so you need to expect at least nine to twelve months before you're ready to get your body back in line again. Nine months, not nine weeks. Take your time and focus on keeping yourself healthy and enjoying those moments when your baby is tiny. They get so big so quickly, and before you know it, it's easy to workout with them sitting, watching you, or even have them working out with you. Don't miss these amazing moments and wish you had spent more time in them because you spent those moments in a nervous panic to meet society's expectations of you as quickly as possible.

Are you happy with yourself most of the time? Are you free of major health concerns? Then the rest will come. Stress makes it harder to lose weight, so don't stress about higher numbers on the scale and unintentionally make your new weight goals even harder than they have to be.

During my postpregnancy recovery on one of my more sad and hopeless days, I thought of this meme: a photo of Jesus with His arms stretched wide and the words "the last time a man gave up anything for his family" written across the bottom. And then I never put it anywhere because I knew my husband would be upset and that it wasn't a true reflection of what my husband does for our family. Even though I have a *great* husband, you can still feel this way. As a new mom, there's a never-ending pressure coming from society on an asinine number of things. Half the people you'll talk to think you should quit your job and be a full-time parent, and the other half want you not to quit your job and make parenting and a career work or maybe there's even pressure to balance a part-time without letting your family needs fall behind. There's pressure to give and give and give of your body until it doesn't even feel like yours anymore, and then after you feel like you've given more than your body has to offer, there's the pressure to get your body looking back to society's standards all because you and your spouse wanted a child. It can feel very single-sided sometimes, like a class project you ended up doing 99 percent of the work for, but it's not your spouse's fault.

If you're in a heterosexual relationship, your partner cannot possibly do the work for you instead. They have certain parts, and you have certain parts, and unfortunately, you get the crap end of the stick on this one. *But* you also got all those early bonding moments with your baby in your belly that your spouse will never have. It's really easy to get caught in the "I'm exhausted, and I'm pulling most of the weight with this baby," but your spouse is, or should be, doing what they can. There are bottles and pump parts that show up clean every day, there's food in the fridge and toilet paper on the roll, the house is clean (enough), and they'll do what they can to take care of the baby when you aren't. Yes, it's a very frustrating time for you, but it's also frustrating for your spouse to see you in so much pain and know they can't do anything to switch places with you. Have patience with them and make sure you're being vocal on the things they can help you with instead of trying to be supermom by yourself.

Parenting is not fifty-fifty. I hope you understood that before you embarked on this journey. Some days, you'll do more than your spouse; some days, they'll do more than you; and some days, read this slowly because it's *very* important, the effort level combined from the two of you won't equal 100 percent. You can only give what you have, so if you and your spouse are so utterly exhausted you only have 40 percent and 50 percent in you that day, then that's what your family will get, *and they'll survive*, and most importantly, *so will you* by not trying to give the extra 10 percent that you don't have.

If your baby will suck a binky/watch TV/eat a pumped/formula bottle as opposed to breastfeeding on days that doing things like entertaining them or pumping/breastfeeding feels like it's going to absolutely kill you, don't do it. Allow yourself the grace to be a little less than your normal that day so you can recover and be better tomorrow. As a society, we put so much pressure on parents to do it all and to do it all "the right way" for fear of messing up your child for life, but no one ever takes into consideration the balancing act of the baby's life and the parents. You can only go so hard and fast for so long before burning out, so if it's a burnout day and no help is on the way and your baby is safe and fed, do what you can to make that day easier on yourself and survive to be a better parent tomorrow.

Happy spouse, happy house. Yes, you guys can do this and learn how to move forward in your new lifestyle. You just need to give yourselves time to adjust to your new normal, and you need to be patient and understanding with your baby and spouse while you do. To get to a more normal ground, you need to release your emotions as they're occurring, which means if you're not having conversations with your spouse when emotions occur even though they suck, you need to have those fights to get to the other side in a good place. Having a baby can put a lot of strain on a marriage, so make sure you find time to not only talk to your spouse but to also have time with just the two of you as well. Let your village of helpers watch your baby and go out to dinner so you can talk without the added pressure of catering to the baby's constant needs. Once you have established a bedtime that the baby sticks to, this becomes significantly easier, but until then, find ways to squeeze in some alone time. Being a parent made me a *much* better communicator because I no longer had the option to let things slide. I needed to make talking about things that bother me a priority so I could get the help I needed.

Bladder incontinence and normalcy (yeah! I can sleep three hours without peeing again)! Leakage is totally normal while your body recovers from having a baby. If it lasts until your six-week appointment, you can always talk to your doctor about seeing a pelvic floor therapist. Whatever you do, *do not* let anyone tell you it's just normal to leak for the rest of your life now. It is not, and you do not have to live like that. Make the appointments and take the time to get your body back to normal so every time you sneeze, you're not reminded that you have had a child. If you don't have the health insurance coverage to go to physical therapy, at the very least, try looking up pelvic floor exercises online and following women on social media who are well-verse in postpartum recovery. There's a lot of free information at your fingertips. A word of forewarning, pelvic floor therapy can include a trained professional sticking their hands in your vagina and/or anus. If you're not comfortable with that, they can help you with exercises only; however, I didn't even know that was something to expect to be asked about at my consultation, so now you know.

Audiobooks, TV series, and e-books are a great way to keep you distracted or let yourself relax while your hands are full of baby, especially in the first few weeks. They'll want to eat so frequently or be held so much that you have a good chunk of time you can commit to those kinds of things. The problem is you usually don't think you'll be stuck until you're already stuck, so keeping a phone with apps for e-books, audiobooks, and TV series already programmed on it in your pocket is a great way to have whatever you need or want at your fingertips, regardless of where you get stuck with or under the baby. I'd recommend a good set of Bluetooth earbuds as well; that way, when your baby is older and easily distracted and they nap on your chest or eat, you still have something you can do without waiting for them to finish what they're doing without risking distracting them from their task.

Your baby should be in extra layers for napping; a sleep sack is an excellent choice once they're past swaddling age. In my experience, it helps them nap longer and lets you get other things done or take a nap. Don't fret if your baby doesn't take to solo naps right away. My son was a contact napper only for six months, but he got there eventually, and it allowed me to get a little more rest during those first few months postpartum, which, looking back, was needed. The contact naps also got him into the habit of taking a longer afternoon nap that translated well to when he was taking naps by himself and let me work some hours for my job, write this book, and clean up the house, so it all worked out in the end. But being "stuck" holding the baby when you have so much to do can be frustrating and sometimes anxiety-inducing if you feel like you're losing too much time in your day. Take deep breaths and try to rest to get some recovery, even if you can't sleep, and remember, this won't last forever, and you have a team of support that can help you if you get really behind.

Your house is fuller than it's ever been as your family expands, and there's more noise and things to do than ever before, but sometimes, you'll be in a house full of things to do and noise with a husband and baby, but you still feel lonely going through this recovery experience by yourself. As supportive and sympathetic as your husband is, he can never empathize with you. He'll never be able to be in the exact same space you were and feel what you're going through mentally and physically with recovery.

Recovery and childbirth are so different for everyone that even mom to mom, the experience is still incredibly different. It's hard with certain topics to feel like you're being heard and understood in your recovery and new position as a mother, and that can make you retreat within yourself. Make sure you're always open with your husband about how you feel, and if they start to say things like "that can't be right," "you're being dramatic," and "I read once that mom's actually feel like…," it's completely fine to shut them down and remind them that your emotions are *valid*. You're allowed to and need to be able to feel, process, and express what you're feeling in all these moments. The second you start to shut down and internalize everything, it becomes a lot harder to have open conversations because now there's even more you need to explain just to get to a basic level of understanding.

Your husband may be getting up to change and sooth the baby and refill your water before you feed them, but when they try to go back to sleep thinking they did all they could, you can still feel very alone feeding your baby and putting them back to sleep. Talk it through with your spouse; maybe have them sit up with you on the worst nights or listen to an audiobook/TV show while you feed your baby. Make sure you're getting the attention you need to feel like this is a team effort and not a solo mission.

Parenting is like babysitting all the time, but the stakes are higher since you can't hand them back at the end of the night. You're constantly thinking, *What can I do to keep them entertained? When do I need to feed them? Where do I put this outfit they pooped all over? Can they eat solid foods yet? Why are they looking at me like that? Am I the entertainment now? Why can't they just sit and play nicely while I read?* And on and on it goes. Mom groups and library programs are great ways to, one, occupy your child and, two, meet other parents and learn some of their tricks without having to come up with them yourself. Anything you can do to interact with parents and children older than your child is an easy way to gain parenting hacks without spending so much time online after your baby goes to sleep.

You're going to have lots of new separation firsts with your baby that can cause parents some anxiety. You'll leave them alone with your husband to go to your six-week appointment, you'll put them in their new room, you'll let them cry themselves to sleep, you'll leave them with someone else to go out alone with your husband, or you'll have a million other situations pop up. It's a hard thing to do, and there are always things in the back of your head that try to convince you that you need to be the person there with your baby at all times, but you need that break to be a better, kinder, more understanding parent. The first time you leave them with someone else, pick the best person you can think of and make sure you go at least thirty minutes away from your house. Drive far enough that if you decide you want to go back to check on them, you know you'll be ending the night early.

Learn how to do things with your baby, jump over that learning curve, and strap them to your chest or put them in a stroller. Another phase of your life begins when you can start doing things *with* your baby instead of waiting for someone else to be able to watch them. Put them in a chest carrier and go to the grocery store, put them in a baby rocker and bring them outside while you garden, put them in a playpen while you work out, let them bounce in a JumpaRoo while you empty the dishwasher and make dinner, or strap them to your back and go to a beer festival. They're going to cry sometimes, but as they learn to listen, talking to them will help decrease their crying. Putting on music while you do other things can help as well. Keep your baby in sight, not only so you can make sure they're still doing well but also so you give them something to watch that keeps their focus and occupies them.

Prepare yourself for your child's one-year shots. I know what you're thinking, *One year? I had to do all the shots leading up to one year. I'm a pro by now.* Trust me you absolutely are not. By one year, your child is just old enough to know you usually protect them and that they're getting hurt by something that isn't them. The one-year shot is when your child looks into your soul, and you can see them thinking, *Why are you holding me down while they hurt me?* And it breaks your heart. I did fine with all of the shots up to one year and then was holding back tears trying to comfort my child for his one-year shots. I could see the hurt and confusion in his face, and for three days afterward, he would cry any time I held him. It was not a fun time, and there's no way to explain to them that you are protecting them, just in a different way than usual. As much as it sucks, you're going to need to do things for them or to them that they won't understand, and they're going to get mad at you with their developing personality, and as much as you're going to want to go cry in the other room every time they look at you and cry, they'll forgive you eventually. You just have to be strong until they do.

Decision burnout is no joke. You go from needing to worry about only you, to worrying about how to take care of yourself and your baby during pregnancy, to making every decision for you, and most if not all of them for your child once they're born. There are food and clothing decisions, schedule decisions, and development decisions when they're very young. Then as they get older, you add in what to make them for each meal, who to interact with, and what they should do every day. It's exhausting, and by the time you've made all those decisions throughout the day, you have no mental power left to dedicate to deciding what you want to do with your time at night so you *waste* it by scrolling through your phone or just sitting staring at the wall, and then you're mad at yourself later for wasting what little free time you had.

Find ways to reduce the number of decisions you make in a week. Developing a weekly schedule that you can use on repeat really helps. If you don't want things to become so programmed, you can write different lists of activities, clothes, foods, etc. that you use a dice or random number generator to make your decisions for the day. I use a combination of the two. Mondays and Thursdays are our library days where we go to the library program, and then the rest of the week, I leave free to play with moms in the area, have some quiet development time, or leave for the two of us to bond so it's not the same thing every week. I've organized his clothes into different types of clothes in each drawer so I have to decide what type of clothing he needs (e.g., PJs, winter clothing, summer clothing), and then I just pick whatever is on top of the pile if it doesn't matter which outfit he wears that day. When I put the laundry away, the clothes I'm putting away go on the bottom of the piles of clothing so his outfits rotate, and I don't have to put much thought into his selections. I meal prep on the weekends and put portioned meals into small Tupperware so all I need to do is shove my hand in the fridge and grab the first thing I touch for a breakfast, snack, or meal option and not decide what to feed him five times a day. You'll find tricks that work for you, but the more mental load you can transfer to your partner so you're sharing the load or making it automated, the less energy you'll need to spend making those decisions every day.

Finding and spending time for yourself when the other people in your family are awake or doing things can feel selfish sometimes. You start working out, reading, or meditating and a million things pop into your head that you need to do or you hear your kid scream-ing and feel the need to intervene, or you hear your kid laughing and want to be a part of their joy, and your brain won't allow you to focus on what you want or need to do to relax. As a result, a lot of the time, you don't start to relax until everything has been done for the day, and your kids are asleep, at which time you're so exhausted that you don't really have the energy to invest in yourself so you don't. Your hobbies go undeveloped, the messages you used to send to friends dwindle to a trickle, and you feel unaccomplished in the things that used to be important to you. As difficult as it may be to take a step back and enjoy time to yourself if you consistently push your needs and development off, it'll show in the way you behave and your interactions with your family. Reroute your thinking until you can believe that this time is a priority and developing yourself is a valuable way to spend your time.

You've put so much time and effort into making your household the way you want it to be. Then you finally get to grow the family you want to fill your house with, and the pretty house you spent so much time developing now becomes a major mess. All your decor needs to get hidden away so your toddling tot won't break things or hurt themselves. Things that were prettily placed in rooms need to now get shoved against the wall so they can be anchored there. Minimalism becomes your new decor profile, and you can no longer pick up pretty random things on shopping trips because if you put it somewhere, your child will inevitably eat it, break it, or hurt themselves with it. There's no winning, and your house is no longer the pretty house you envisioned having. Toys scatter the floors, and just when you thought your day was as bad as it was going to get, you inevitably step on the sharpest toy your child owns and immediately fly off the handle. Then you calm down, and you're mad at yourself for yelling at your kid to clean up their mess, or you're upset with how many cuss words you just dropped in front of them in a thirty-second window.

The more kids you have the longer, this window drags out, but eventually they stop putting things in their mouths and destroying things you want to decorate with, and you can start making decorations with them and enjoying the creations you make becoming your decor. Then when you finally can get your house back to the prettily decorated home you imagined, you start to miss the finger paint artwork on the fridge and the toilet paper roll pumpkin they made you. The only advice I have for your decor for the time being is to find a way to put it up high before it goes out of fashion hiding in your storage room for the next ten years.

Appendix 1

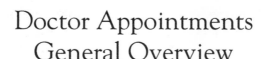

Doctor Appointments General Overview

When I first found out I was pregnant, I was shocked to find out my doctor wouldn't immediately book me an appointment, and you'll see a lot of other moms in appendix 2 felt the same way. I had to wait until eight to ten weeks after my last period for my first appointment. Since I knew I was pregnant three weeks past my last period, I felt like I was waiting forever and was already messing up my child by not seeing a doctor immediately. I made my appointment for the first day of week eight and waited impatiently to see the doctor, who ended up actually being a nurse practitioner. I peed in a cup when we got there, they took my weight, we talked to the nurse, I had a transvaginal ultrasound done to confirm the pregnancy, they drew some bloodwork, I was given a packet of information, and they sent me on my way, telling me to come back every four weeks until I was twenty-eight weeks pregnant.

If you are given a packet of information, I'd suggest reading it *very closely* and going back to it at least once a trimester, but I'd recommend initially before every doctor's appointment. There was a lot of information in my packet that the doctors and nurses didn't seem to feel the need to tell me in person unless I asked them specific questions on an item. They expect you to know this packet very thoroughly if you want any idea about what to expect during the time you'll spend at their office.

After your twenty-eighth-week appointment, you'll switch to biweekly appointments until thirty-six weeks, then from thirty-six weeks until delivery, you'll be going to the doctors once a week for a checkup. Each appointment included a urine culture (peeing in a cup), weight check, consultation with the physician, a doppler reading of the baby's heart rate (unless you were having an ultrasound done that day), and some prodding of the stomach to see how much your uterus was growing. I assume all doctor's offices are slightly different in their timing, but below is a general timeline for the different shots/test/items that were done or needed by me during my pregnancy.

An item with an * is invasive, an item with a ~ is a shot or blood work, and an item with a ° is noninvasive and is either a drink, pelvic ultrasound, or peeing in a cup. I'll go over a basic description of what the tests accomplish at the bottom of the outline, but there is a lot of additional information online if you have deeper questions.

Week of Pregnancy	Testing Done
Week 8-First Visit	Routine blood work~, transvaginal ultrasound*, and urine testing°
Week 12	Noninvasive prenatal testing (NIPT)*, first trimester screen (FTS)*, and urine test°
Week 16	Alpha-fetoprotein (AFP) test~ and urine test°
Week 20	Full body scan ultrasound of the baby° and urine test°
Week 24	Urine test° and one-hour glucose test°~
Week 25	Three-hour glucose test°~ (if applicable)
Week 28	Flu shot~, T-dap~, and RhoGAM~ (if applicable)
Weeks 30–34	Urine test

Week 35	Urine test,° strep B culture*, and COVID-19 booster*
Week 36	·Urine test° and US Department of Labor Family Medical Leave Act (FMLA) paperwork°
Weeks 38–40+	Urine test° and dilation checks* (if you consent)

But what does it all mean?

I've included some information on the tests listed above from a basic point of view:

- ❖ *Routine blood work*—The initial blood work test is used to check for preexisting diseases and conditions and to confirm the blood type of the mother.
- ❖ *NIPT*—Samples of your blood are taken to capture parts of the baby's DNA from the placenta. (Cool!) This is a screen for chromosomes 13 (Patau syndrome), 18 (Edwards syndrome), and 21 (Down's syndrome).
- ❖ *FTS*—This is also a screen for chromosomes 13, 18, and 21; however, this also includes an ultrasound to measure the baby's neck and see if they have a nose. Blood is taken to check for the PAPP-A and hCG. I had the blood work done at the FTS appointment but then did not have the ultrasound part completed until the twenty-week body scan. All of the information the doctors will collect is then used to calculate the overall risk your child has of birth defects.
- ❖ *AFP*—This blood test screens for neural tube defects.
- ❖ *Full body scan*—You'll be getting an external (pelvic) ultrasound where they'll make sure the baby has developed the proper number of body parts, and they'll see what the growth of the baby puts the estimated conception and delivery date at. Something I did not know is the estimate delivery date doesn't usually change your actual due date

estimate; it's more just a reflection of how big the baby is at the time. Only in some extreme situations will the doctor choose to change the estimated due date in your charts. My son measured big my entire pregnancy, so we always had an earlier due date than the forty-week period, and he waited forty-one and a half weeks to come.

❖ *One-hour glucose test*—You'll get some blood work done as a starting point to see where your blood sugar levels are. You'll chug a very sugary drink, and you'll wait an hour and get more blood work done. They're looking to see how your body processes sugars and if it can do it in an appropriate amount of time. You cannot drink during this test (even water), and they recommend no carbs or sugars before you have the test, so try to schedule this first thing in the morning.

❖ *Three-hour glucose test*—If you fail the one-hour glucose test, they'll make you do a three-hour test. It's the same as the one-hour except at hour two and three, you also get blood work done, so there are four points of measurement to look at: predrink, one hour after drink, two hours after drink, and three hours after drink.

❖ *Flu shot*—This shot helps protect you from getting the flu during your pregnancy. You'll get this shot whenever the season starts (usually September) during your pregnancy. It's a good idea to have your spouse and anyone who will be around the baby right after birth get this vaccine as well.

❖ *Tdap*—This is one shot that covers you from tetanus, diphtheria, and pertussis (whooping cough). It's a good idea to have your spouse and anyone who will be around the baby right after birth get this vaccine as well.

❖ *RhoGAM*—If you have a negative blood type, you will get this shot. It's easy to test the mother's blood type and harder to test the baby's, so every woman with a negative blood type receives this shot. In the case of a mom having a negative blood type and the baby having a positive blood type, your body can develop Rh antibodies, which would start to attack the positive blood type. You'll also get one of these after delivery as well.

❖ *COVID-19 booster*—This shot helps build your immunity to the COVID-19 virus. It's a good idea to have your spouse and anyone who will be around the baby right after birth get this vaccine as well. If you haven't gotten a first shot of the vaccine, you'll have to get a few shots in a row to be considered fully vaccinated, so the sooner you start, the better.

❖ *Strep B*—This is a vaginal swab test to make sure you don't have Group B streptococcus bacteria before delivery. If your test comes back positive, they'll put you on antibiotics during labor to make sure your baby doesn't get it.

❖ *FMLA paperwork*—If you're going back to work after your baby and you want your job secured and to be able to use any benefits from the company you work for, you need to get your FMLA paperwork filled out by the doctor before you go on leave.

❖ *Dilation checks*—This is invasive and involves the doctor sticking their fingers into the opening of your cervix to see if you've begun dilating. You can have this checked after the thirty-eight-week appointment, or you don't have to have it checked. The theory is knowing if your dilated can help you know how far your body is progressing and if you're getting close to ready to delivery. In practice, though, each person progresses so differently that they're not a great metric. Just because you're three centimeters dilated this week doesn't mean you'll be six centimeters by next week or that you'll make any progress at all. These are slightly painful since the doctors have to reach their fingers so far up into you to touch your cervix, so after I had the first one and I knew I was slightly dilated, I declined having any others, except for when we were in the hospital getting ready to deliver my baby because then they need to know.

Initial packet of information provided by my OB that you should ask for from yours:

- ❖ Emergency numbers
- ❖ Prenatal basic care
- ❖ Safe over-the-counter medicines
- ❖ What to watch for in each trimester
- ❖ Weight gain guidelines during pregnancy
- ❖ Environmental hazards to avoid
- ❖ Pregnancy resources
- ❖ Nutrition demand changes during pregnancy

Appendix 2

Real Stories from Real Moms

Here are some interview questions from five moms, all to show even the same woman can have completely different childbirth experiences. Hopefully, these stories will give you a little insight into what to potentially expect during the leaving for, birthing, and postpartum experience, as well as be a good reminder for how plans can change.

Mom 1

1) What were your expectations on pregnancy and the process before going to your first doctor's appointment? Were you happy with the care you received, or did you feel like you weren't properly prepared for what to expect throughout the process?

   To back up, before I was pregnant, at my last well woman's exam, before we decided to have a baby, I asked about what I'd need to do to prep my body to get ready to have a child. I brought all my vitamins and supplements with me to make sure they'd give the baby everything it needed to grow healthy, and the doctor told me as long as I'd been taking those for three months, we could start trying, and everything would be good. I remember sitting there, looking at the door. The doctor had just left, and I was in shock. She didn't want me to take an IQ test? No one needed to come look at my house to see if we could provide a good home for a baby? No one did a background or finance check on my husband and me? Don't get me wrong, I'd have been mad if they told me I needed to do those things, but it felt like an underwhelmingly small list of things to do to have a child.

I found out I was pregnant at three weeks, so I hadn't even missed a period yet, but I knew my body enough to know, and turned out, I was right. I called my OB the same day I took my pregnancy test and was panicked to hear I'd have to wait until eight to ten weeks for an appointment. Didn't they know I had no clue what I was doing and needed an expert's advice on how to do everything I possibly could to have a healthy baby? I even asked if they had a welcome packet I could get early to start reading up on information, and they *assured me* (I promise it was not reassuring) I'd get all that information at the first appointment.

The rest of my care felt the same way. I'd show up to my appointment having no clue what to expect to happen to me that day or what they'd need. Until I got to the end of my pregnancy and was meeting with the doctors at every appointment, I felt like I never knew which way was up. Even when I was meeting with the doctors, I still didn't know what to expect for each visit, and I felt like there was "nothing they could do" for my pain or concerns, but they at least were able to explain what was happening to my body in a scientific manner, and that put me more at ease.

2) Did you feel like your concerns were adequately heard or did you feel like anything you brought up was always pushed off in a "you're pregnant you're going to be uncomfortable" category?

During appointments, I felt like the first question from the nurse practitioners was always "How are you feeling?" and then as soon as I'd tell them, they'd tell me that was expected and wouldn't give me any solutions to lessen my pain or any research to back up their "this is normal" claim, which left me feeling like I wasn't very heard during my pregnancy. Looking back, because I felt like I wasn't very supported by my OB staff, I feel like I went overboard and did way more research on way more topics than I needed to. Without doing research, I felt like I didn't know what type of questions to ask and felt like I wasn't getting anything out of my checkups, so I feel like I flipped to the opposite extreme and started looking into things almost too much.

3) What was your birthing plan before you went to the hospital and how did it differ from what you experienced?

My birthing plan included having a doula come to our house once my labor started, laboring at home until I had to go to the hospital, trying to do things without medication (but understanding if things changed the day of), being up and mobile for as long as possible, and having a vaginal birth. What actually happened was my baby decided he was too comfortable and did not want to leave, so I needed an induction. With my long labor, I ended up getting an epidural per my doula's recommendation. Since my water broke during my first contraction and I thought my baby kicked a contraction, I immediately *thought* there was absolutely no reason to feel that all night. Thankfully, I was still able to have a vaginal birth, but my baby turned at the last minute, so we ended up needing to use forceps to get him out.

4) Did you falsely think you were going into labor at any time during the pregnancy? What was that phone call with the doctor/experience like?

I thought my water broke a few days after my due date. I took a bath and then showered, and I guess some water from the bath ended up getting sucked up in there because halfway through my shower, I felt it trickle down my leg. I texted our doula to see if she thought it was my water breaking, did some googling, and eventually called the doctor. The doctor on call at the time told me he didn't think my water had broken, but if I wanted to be safe, I could come into the hospital and have it checked. I'm a very risk adverse person, and I hadn't felt like anyone really knew for sure, so we decided to go in and have it checked. My water had not broken, but we still went through all the testing to be sure.

When we arrived, we went into the labor and delivery department's triage area. I peed in a cup and got changed into a hospital gown. All my vitals were taken, and they stuck this incredibly dry swab into my vagina to let it sit there for a minute. That didn't feel great. It was like having a too large size of a tampon inserted, not because the swab was that big but because I felt like it was trying to suck up more liquid than was in my vagina. After the swab determined my water hadn't broken, the nurse called the doctor to update him, and he released us via the phone call. I got dressed, and we went home. We had to deal with a little disappointment that night since we didn't get to meet our baby, but we were glad we got it checked, and the induction date was close enough at that point that we knew it wouldn't be too much longer before we met our baby anyways.

5) Can you describe how you went into labor and the steps from when you thought you were going into labor until you had your baby in your arms?

I needed an induction since my son was too cozy in the womb. That means the doctor's office scheduled a day I'd call the hospital and ask them what time they wanted me to come in. Based off their availability, they'd tell me what time we needed to be at the hospital to begin the induction process. I was supposed to call the hospital the morning of the induction at 9:30 a.m., and they'd tell me what time to come in. Instead, I woke up to a missed call from the hospital at 6:30 a.m. and was stressed when I called them back. Thankfully, they hadn't given up my spot to the next caller in-line and asked me to come in as soon as we could. So I woke up my husband, showered, and ate breakfast, and we threw our bags in the car and left. We kept our doula up to date but didn't feel the need for her to come in at the time since we didn't know how long the induction would take. Once we got to the front desk and were checked in, I was forced (company policy) into a wheelchair to be carted off to the labor and delivery wing. I was taken to the room I'd have my baby in and met with the doctor on call and our nurse.

The doctor checked how far dilated I was and explained she thought the best way to induce the delivery would be Pitocin, but she listened to the other inductions methods I had researched and answered all my questions before I decided she was right, and Pitocin would be the best and straightest path forward. What I didn't know when I'd been doing research was a lot of the other dilation methods only get you so far, and a lot of the time, you still need Pitocin at the end, if you haven't begun dilating much before you're induced, so I figured if I'd need it at some point we might as well just use that method for the whole process. The nurse started me on an IV drip, read my initial vital signs, and gave me the first dose of Pitocin.

The hospital mobile baby heart monitors were broken, so I had to stay within six feet of my bed any time I had to be attached to the monitors. Once the Pitocin started, I spent the first two hours on the monitor, and then as long as our son's heart rate stayed strong and consistent, I could get off the monitor for two hours and walk around. I spent the first two hours watching a movie and afterward was cleared to walk around for two hours. The hospital had a pregnancy trail that was a series of walkways and paths they allowed you to walk that were supposed to help you induce yourself.

I was on Pitocin for fifteen hours before my water broke. It took me a minute to realize what was happening. I thought my son had kicked a contraction at first and then, a few seconds later, felt like I needed to pee, but by the time I got up to pee, there was water everywhere. The overall process was taking so long that my doula recommended I get an epidural so I could sleep through the night, so as soon as my water broke, I asked for my epidural. It took about thirty minutes for the anesthesiologist to show up, but since my water had broken in bed and we had to clean the bed and myself up, it felt like five minutes. By the time my epidural was done, it was already after midnight, so I tried to sleep/rest on and off. The second-shift nurse was in and out all night, checking on me and adjusting the heart rate monitors. Around 9:30 a.m., the doctor came in and told me I could start pushing. I changed nurses one more time, and the next doctor started their shift before I started pushing.

Because of the epidural, I couldn't feel my legs at all, so my doula and a nurse held my legs. I was lucky in that the nurse for this shift was training a nurse that was new to their hospital, so I had one nurse to watch the overall progression and one to hold my leg so my husband could be by my head instead of holding a leg. The epidural left me completely numb, so I didn't have any indication on when I should push. The nurse would watch the monitor to see when a contraction was starting, and we'd begin the pushing process. I wasn't very impressed with the nurses' instructions on pushing. They just told me to "push how it feels right," but my epidural had given me no feeling at all below my bra line, so I didn't feel any indication I should push, let alone something in one specific area.

At each contraction, I'd sit up, hold my breath, and push for ten seconds. We'd do that three times and then wait for the next contraction to try again. The doctor came in after three hours of pushing to see if I wanted to keep going or if I thought we'd need to use a vacuum or forceps or do a C-section. I told him I wanted to keep going and pushed for another two hours. He had instructed me to try and push form my abdomen down, and I felt like that was helpful advice, and we finally started progressing after that.

At the very end, my son turned; and because of the position of his head, we had to use forceps to get him out. The doctor had explained to me what each option (vacuum, forceps, and C-section) would look like when he came in at three hours, so, thankfully, I had some time to absorb what those were before being told my option was forceps or a vacuum for delivery at this point. I asked him which he thought was safer for the baby and I, and he said forceps (which are essentially giant metal salad tongs). So a NICU team was assembled in the room, and the doctor used forceps to remove my baby.

I couldn't see the delivery of my baby since the doctor moved the mirror out of the way to use the forceps. My husband could see everything, though, and it really freaked him out. Our baby had a very coned head when he was born and didn't immediately cry, so my husband thought we had lost the baby during delivery and was devastated. Immediately after delivery, my son was checked on by the NICU team. While he was being checked on, my doctor was sewing me up. I couldn't see my baby even though he was essentially beside me because the team of nurses was so large. My husband was able to go around the corner and get a look at him from the front. Once he could see our son and hear him crying, my husband realized he was fine, and the relief was so sudden he felt lightheaded and had to sit down for a little. When our baby was all cleaned up and had a hat and diaper on, the nurses brought him back over to me and laid him on my chest so I could hold him. He was nuzzled up so far to my neck I felt like I didn't actually get to see him at first. I just held him close and was thankful he was finally here and healthy.

6) Can you describe your postdelivery experience at the hospital? Please include your experience with breastfeeding, your body's experience in postdelivery feelings, what the nurses helped with and where you wish they supported you more, where your baby was, and how long you stayed at the hospital.

After receiving and holding my son for a few minutes, my stitches were finished, and we talked to the doctor for a while. I was starving, so I asked the nurses if I could eat anything. I ate a protein bar we had brought while they worked on getting me a meal, and a pediatrician came in to check on our son. While our son was being evaluated, I came down *very hard* off the epidural. It was to the point where I was in so much pain I was throwing up and felt like I couldn't see people's faces. As a result, I was given some morphine. I'm unsure if it was the morphine or the pain, but I get things in flashes after that for a bit. Because I didn't feel like I could safely hold my son, my husband held him the whole time we were in the delivery room. While I was trying to manage my pain, my husband took his shirt off and did skin to skin with our son so he could still get some parental bonding.

While I was trying to recover so we could move to the recovery unit, out of nowhere, I felt like I had to pee so badly my bladder was going to explode. The nurses brought a bedpan over to me. They helped lift my body to sit on top of the bedpan and told me to pee, but it was a really awkward setup, and regardless of how hard I tried, I could not find the muscles to do it. They eventually gave up and gave me a catheter but told me once they catheterize someone after the procedure, they're not allowed to do it for another twelve hours, so I had to learn to find those muscles quickly. We moved into the recovery room after that. They put me in a wheelchair and the baby in a rolling cart, and a nurse pushed me while my husband pushed our son behind me until we got to the room. I was still in and out during this process. I don't remember any of the lactation consultant's advice. I just remember telling her to do what she needed to do and lying in the bed with my nipples out, struggling to stay awake and trying to listen.

I was brought dinner and was coming back enough that I was able to eat something and keep it down this time. The first recovery nurse I had was *amazing* and helped get me to the bathroom and relearn how to pee since my body somehow managed to forget how to do that between induction and delivery. She taught me how to take care of my stitches area and showed me how to make the pad/underwear combo I used the whole time I was at the hospital to cool and heal my stitches. She gave our baby a bath and, when we looked utterly exhausted, offered to take our son to the nursery. I wasn't sure how I felt about my son being out of our sight for any period of time. The nurse could see me hesitating and told me she didn't have to take him but that not all nurses will offer or agree to take the babies to the nursery and she only had a few more hours left in her shift. Out of utter exhaustion, we eventually agreed to let her take our son to the nursery, and my husband and I instantly fell asleep until she brought him back.

Our recovery time in the hospital that first night was a little overwhelming. I didn't expect my muscles to hurt so badly, and I really didn't expect my husband to have no clue how to do anything related to our baby. I hadn't taken into account, before we got to the hospital, that he had never babysat growing up, and he didn't have nieces or nephews, so he had no clue how to sooth a baby or even change it. Looking back, I really should have explained some general care to him before delivery so I could lay in bed and recover a little more, as opposed to teaching him how to do things in the hospital.

The first night in the hospital was very hard. Because I had been so out of it when the lactation consultant was explaining how to breastfeed, I didn't learn anything about the process, which might not have been a problem if they had a consultant that worked nights, but they didn't, so by the time I realized I needed the lactation consultant again, they were gone, and I was in a panic about how to feed my baby. The nurse on shift tried to help me breastfeed, and when my son still wasn't getting anything and self-expression wasn't working, she brought in a pump for me to try and pump some colostrum that I could then feed our baby with a gloved finger. It was very stress-inducing, and I left what felt like a million messages for the lactation consultant, asking her to come to our room the second she was back on-site.

My family came the next day to visit us and meet our baby, and it was nice to have some normalcy thrown into what was a completely new experience. It gave us some time to sit and not have to worry about holding the baby since my family was very excited to get to hold him. The doctor came in to check on me while my sister and brother-in-law were visiting and gave me some general care instructions for at home and major signs to look out for to call the hospital. There were tons of people in and out all day to test the baby and check on me and him. I wasn't prepared for how little sleep you get after having a baby, and by the time we left on the fourth day (second full day after delivery), I was exhausted and ready for a major night's rest...which isn't really a thing with a three-day-old. I wish I had my family come visit for the first week to take care of our son during the day so we could sleep. I think I would have recovered significantly faster if I had.

7) Can you describe your physical recovery experience at home and how long you worked to recover to "normal" (i.e., did you go to PT, need X-rays, use advice from parents, wing it, do research into how to recover, etc.)?

I was floored by the amount of recovery time my body needed postpartum. I hadn't been prepared for all the different ways my body could need help in the months after my baby was delivered. I felt like I recovered from the vaginal/uterus part of birth pretty quickly and was back up and going on walks within a few weeks. What I was not prepared for was how five hours of pushing and a couple days of sitting all day on my tailbone would wreak havoc on my body. The hospital gave me pretty good instructions on how to take care of my stitches, but the rest was more trial and error for recovery since there weren't many instructions given, and I wasn't in the right mental place to be doing research at the time.

I had really bad tailbone pain after my son was born. We immediately ordered a tailbone donut to sit on and an inflatable donut for my sitz baths, but sleeping on my back and sitting were unbearable, which is really difficult to manage when you're breastfeeding every two to three hours, so you're sitting up to feed your baby, and then in the small windows when you can sleep, you're not sleeping much anyways. I was in so much pain by week 3 that I made an early appointment with my OB, which was not helpful at all. They sent me for an X-ray, and when nothing was found, they told me I was fine, and I'd recover eventually. So three more weeks went by, and I was in for my six-week appointment, also severely underwhelming, and when I told them I still had such terrible tailbone pain I couldn't sit without the donut or sleep, they gave me a referral for physical therapy, which I got put on a two-month waiting list for and then attended for seven months before being cleared for "normal activities," which was still less than my pre-pregnancy level, activity. In addition to the PT, I received a cortisone injection by my tailbone to help manage the pain and was going to the chiropractor twice a week for five months. The chiropractor recommended a few massages a few weeks after birth as well since my muscles were all so tight because I hadn't started PT yet.

Because I pushed for so long, and in what I think was an incorrect manner, since the nurses didn't help much with instructions, I ended up needing a colonoscopy about a month after delivery as well. The prep work sucked. (Seriously, never wipe your butt by the time you take the laxative. It feels like your poop is basically water and salt, so just use your peri bottle, and it'll save you so much pain.) The procedure was relatively easy, and I found out I had some anal fissures and hemorrhoids, but thankfully, nothing that time wouldn't heal.

8) Is there anything else you would like to tell me about your pregnancy?

During my pregnancy, I had done a lot of research on the natural release of chemicals from your body and how certain drugs at the hospital can block the uptake of those chemicals and make you less likely to bond as strongly with your baby. As a result, I went into the birthing process thinking I'd want to do things naturally with no Pitocin and no epidural; however, my baby was very comfortable in the womb and did not want to leave, so I had to have an induction. As seen above, I ended up with the epidural as well. I firmly believe every mother gets to choose to have her baby the way she wants to, but if you're looking for my two cents, I will never, by choice, go through labor without an epidural again. I still was excited to meet my baby and was able to not be in pain during the entire process. I needed stitches through three layers of muscles after my son was born and was glad I didn't have to feel all those muscles ripping before I was numbed to get all the stitches I needed.

Mom 2

1) What were your expectations on pregnancy and the process before going to your first doctor's appointment? Were you happy with the care you received, or did you feel like you weren't properly prepared for what to expect throughout the process?

Backing up to when I first found out I was pregnant, I wasn't sure what to do at all! I thought I would call the doctor, I'd be seen in a couple weeks, and that they would do blood work and confirm my pregnancy. I found out at about three to four weeks pregnant, and when I called, they said, "Oh, we won't see you until eight weeks." I was shocked! So I kept taking test after test to confirm I was still pregnant because I didn't have any symptoms, so I didn't even believe it. After searching Dr. Google, I came to find out that's totally normal not to be seen until eight weeks at least since before then, there is nothing to really see. I also did a lot of prep of "what to expect" for appointments and ways to keep healthy and how to make sure baby was getting good supplements. I wish there would have been something the doctor had told me prior to my eight-week appointment of what exact nutrients a good supplement has (particularly folate being an important one) and things to avoid. All of that didn't come until my first doctor's visit.

When I received care for my first appointment, I was still in Kentucky. The doctors and nurses there were amazing. I did some questions and blood work and a urinalysis to confirm pregnancy, then they did a transvaginal ultrasound to date the pregnancy and give an EDD (estimate due date). I really liked the team there, but it was only for one visit, and then I moved down to South Carolina where my current doctor was. That first appointment there also went really well! We heard our baby's heartbeat and got a full schedule of appointments and things I would need to do visit-wise for my whole pregnancy. I really liked it.

2) Did you feel like your concerns were adequately heard or did you feel like anything you brought up was always pushed off in a "you're pregnant you're going to be uncomfortable" category?

I really liked my doctor a lot because she would always ask me questions to make sure everything was okay. She never dismissed anything I said but would rather answer it and explain that it was normal and that if I was concerned, the office could always be reached, and I could make another appointment to see her. She was great!

One really positive experience I did have, though, was when I had gotten a sinus infection, and I had to call the on-call doctor to confirm I could take a specific antibiotic. They were so understanding of my questions (much more understanding than the urgent care I went to), and they told me to also let my doctor know so she was aware.

3) What was your birthing plan before you went to the hospital and how did it differ from what you experienced?

Oh, man, this is a rough one! So long story short, I'd say my birth experience was a complete 180 of what I thought it was going to be. I didn't have any complications throughout my whole pregnancy. My son had been head down, and I was prepared to try a natural birth for as long as possible and get an epidural if I wanted, but I was anticipating a vaginal birth. What I did not expect was to run into some roadblocks along the way and how the course of action I took might have increased the chance of my unplanned C-section.

When I got admitted at 6:00 a.m., I was immediately put on an IV and a Pitocin drip as my contractions hadn't picked up since my water broke at 11:00 p.m. the previous night. I was dilated to about three centimeters when I wanted the epidural. The nurses told me it would take anywhere to thirty minutes to one hour to get the epidural, so I told them a bit earlier that I wanted it. Well, this was roadblock 1. Not only did I have to get this epidural alone (just me, the nurse, and the anesthesiologist) but it also caused my blood pressure to drop drastically and caused my son's heart rate to drop too with each contraction I had. Ultimately, when they stopped the Pitocin, my contractions stopped, and he was fine, but it also caused him to move back up the birth canal.

I labored like that until about 9:30 p.m. when my doctor had a serious talk with me about her concerns. She did not want to do a C-section, but she also mentioned if I kept going further, it might have turned into an emergency, and that would have been even worse. After some talking and tears, my husband and I decided this was the best decision for my son and me. This was a terrifying moment because this was something my husband and I did not prepare for *at all*. I was honestly so numb through it all. I was sleepy, I was thirsty, and I felt like I was living outside of my body for that moment in time. I slept through almost the whole procedure, so I didn't pass out on the OR table, and thankfully, my doctor had everyone leave me be so I could close my eyes. Right before the baby came out, my husband came in and got to see his baby be born, and then I saw our little bean—he was so squishy and looked like a little alien, but I loved him!

After delivery, I was wheeled to post op. This was the worst of it all because I was there for an hour, just me and two nurses, while they massaged my uterus every fifteen minutes. I didn't get to hold my baby or see him nor my husband for the first hour and a half after I had my son. I kept asking questions about recovery and all that, and the nurses just said, "Oh, you'll find out when you get to the next room." I was shocked that I wasn't able to see my baby or my husband, but quite frankly, I was just numb at that point. Everything I had originally thought would happen in my head was nothing like I actually experienced.

4) Did you falsely think you were going into labor at any time during the pregnancy? What was that phone call with the doctor/experience like?

The only time I thought I was and it turned out to be false was the night my water broke. I thought I had been leaking amniotic fluid all day, so I went into triage, and after some checks and an ultrasound, they said my water didn't break yet and sent me home.

5) Can you describe how you went into labor and the steps from when you thought you were going into labor until you had your baby in your arms?

Two hours after I got discharged from triage (story above), we went to get ice cream, and I took a nice shower. I was just about to crawl into bed when all of a sudden, I felt a gush of fluid. I ran to the toilet, and as soon as I sat down, it gushed again. I laughed and told my husband "you will not believe what just happened," and we both laughed. At that point, I had no contractions at all. When I called the on-call doctor, he told me to wait until 6:00 a.m. the next morning to go in if the contractions didn't get worse before then. At 5:30 a.m. (I was super anxious and excited), we went into triage, and my water definitely had broken, so I was admitted and started on Pitocin because my contractions were barely there.

At about three centimeters, I asked for an epidural, and that process was hard. Per the hospital's policy (which I hadn't asked about previously), I had to be alone. It was me, the nurse, and the anesthesiologist. I had to sit very still and just squeeze a pillow while being poked and prodded. Once it was all done, I was pretty much bedridden and labored with a peanut ball. Right after, around probably 7:00 p.m., my blood pressure dropped drastically, and with every contraction, the baby's heart rate dropped too. That was when they decided to drop the Pitocin, and my son went back to normal. Every time they would try to start it to induce contractions, his heart rate would drop, and they would have to cut it off. That continued on for about two hours when my doctor finally started to think that it would be best to have a C-section before things turned into an emergency.

My husband and I were scared because we had *no* idea what to expect, and it was terrifying knowing I would be going into surgery at that point. I also was starting to have my epidural wear off, so while I was talking with everyone, trying to make a decision, I was shaking, and my teeth were chattering so much that I had to bite on a napkin so they didn't crack! At about 9:30 p.m., I was wheeled back to the OR where they started the procedure. I was so sleepy that my doctor kind of just let me relax and sleep until my husband was brought in to see our son being born. At 10:05 p.m., he was born, and while I got stitched up, my husband got to walk him to the nursery area and see a lot of his firsts and spend that time with him.

6) Can you describe your postdelivery experience at the hospital? Please include your experience with breastfeeding, your body's experience in postdelivery feelings, what the nurses helped with and where you wish they supported you

more, where your baby was, and how long you stayed at the hospital.

My postdelivery was probably some of the worst. Immediately after my C-section, I was wheeled back to this dark area that was *so* quiet where I was kept for the next hour to make sure I wasn't going to hemorrhage. It was me and two nurses who weren't very helpful in answering questions like what recovery would look like, what can I expect while I'm at the hospital recovering, etc. I spent that first hour alone without my husband or our son, and it was the worst. I was crying and shaking, and I just wanted to be with my baby. Once I was wheeled back to the nursery/postdelivery room, that was *so* much better.

Day 2 after surgery was probably the hardest. I was forced to get up and walk and move around, and I decided I wanted a shower as well. I wish the nurses would have been a bit more helpful in terms of helping me get situated in bed, but thankfully, I had my mom and my husband. They helped me so much with my recovery and all the walking and moving. I had to track all my urine output that first day to make sure my bladder was still intact, so that was interesting, and I didn't expect to have to do that. I was also in some pretty intense pain in my neck/clavicle area, which I was told was gas from being cut open. I thought that was so interesting because I didn't know that could happen!

Breastfeeding was a process. When I first got to my son, I latched him on both boobs to see if he would get anything. He didn't get anything as my milk wasn't even close to coming in. The lactation consultant actually came by my room quite often and was really great. She helped me with some tools, figuring out a good latch and position, and how to try to hand express some milk. It was *so* much harder those first few days, and we supplemented with some of the bottles of formula at the hospital. Once my milk came in, there were a few concerns I had about my son getting enough milk because he didn't hit his birth weight until about week 3.

7) Can you describe your physical recovery experience at home and how long you worked to recover to "normal" (i.e., did you go to PT, need X-rays, use advice from parents, wing it, do research into how to recover, etc.)?

I was very fortunate to have a lot of help at home when we were discharged. I had my mom for three straight weeks and then about five days where I was alone before my mother-in-law came for two weeks split up. I had been encouraged by my husband and my mother-in-law to walk around and keep moving to help with my C-section recovery scar. I think that helped a bunch. A main part of my recovery was limited mobility. I was confined to the first floor for about five weeks. I also couldn't drive or lift anything heavier than the baby. My family really was strict on all that, so they did chores, cooked, and took care of the dog while I just took care of the baby and myself. That helped me immensely. I would say by week 4, I felt really good. I still had some numbness on my skin around the scar, but I looked up some Instagram accounts on C-section scar mobility so I could work on trying to get those nerves to regenerate.

One thing in particular I struggled with outside of the physical was my emotions. I did not know and was not expecting to feel so many strong emotions after giving birth. For the first six weeks of my son's life, I cried so much and kept waking up for every noise he made. I honestly thought every noise he made would mean something would go wrong, and he would die. I cried and cried, and finally, at my five- or six-week checkup, my doctor asked about my mental health. She kept kind of prodding to make sure I was telling her everything, and finally, I just burst into tears. I got put on some low-dose medicine to help with PPA, but that saved my sanity and helped me just become so much of a happier mom for my baby.

Mom 3

1) What were your expectations on pregnancy and the process before going to your first doctor's appointment? Were you happy with the care you received, or did you feel like you weren't properly prepared for what to expect throughout the process?

I had all the feelings when I found out I was pregnant, like everyone, I'm sure! I remember calling my ob-gyn immediately after getting my positive test and feeling like I had no idea what I was doing. I informed the receptionist that I got a positive pregnancy test, and I wasn't sure what to do next. She giggled and said we needed to schedule an appointment for ten weeks. I was completely shocked that it was going to be so far out. I asked if I could come in sooner just to make sure everything looked all right and to ease any of my nerves, to which they declined and said to come in if I experienced any bleeding. Ten weeks felt like an eternity, and any little pain made my nerves go through the roof. I wasn't sure if what I was feeling was something normal since I had cramping and breast pain as my body was starting to change. I discovered the What to Expect app, and thankfully, reading testimonies from other women eased my nerves a bit. I wish that my doctor would have brought me in for an early appointment just to explain what's to come, like a "welcome to pregnancy" or "pregnancy 101" crash course since I had never experienced any of that before. I did a lot of research on my own to help prepare myself and felt very nervous going into my first appointment.

2)   Did you feel like your concerns were adequately heard or did you feel like anything you brought up was always pushed off in a "you're pregnant you're going to be uncomfortable" category?

I received a folder of information at my first appointment, which was helpful. At that time, I wasn't really sure what questions to ask. My OB told me everything looked great, and there were no concerns at that time. There were birthing classes available to go over the information in the folder. I attended the first one during my second trimester but didn't feel like I was learning anything new from what I was able to read and research on my own.

Luckily, I didn't have too many issues during my pregnancy, and my midwife was great throughout the journey. Toward the end of my pregnancy, I did have a few episodes of high blood pressure to which my midwife sent me up to the OB floor at the hospital to be monitored for a few hours. I was taken up to the labor and delivery floor at the hospital and placed in the hospital bed. They hooked me up to the fetal monitor around my waist and a blood pressure machine that was recording vitals every fifteen minutes for about an hour. They performed some routine labs to make sure nothing looked alarming and took a urine sample as well. After about an hour of lying in the bed, relaxing, my blood pressure was getting lower, which was communicated with the doctor on call. He allowed me to be released and for me to record my blood pressure at home a few times a day. I also had to do a twenty-four-hour urine collection to evaluate for high protein levels over the next day. Everything ended up looking good with no concerns when I followed up with my doctor the next week. I feel like my midwife aired on the side of caution, as well as the other providers in the medical group.

3) What was your birthing plan before you went to the hospital and how did it differ from what you experienced?

I was very hopeful for having a vaginal delivery at the start of my pregnancy. I was okay with having medication and an epidural if I were to go down that road. At the end of the day, I just wanted a healthy self and baby at the end of the process. I wanted to stay away from a cesarean section if I could because it's a major surgery, and working in the medical field has been a curse and blessing for knowledge about that. I ended up having to undergo a C-section because my son was breeched.

4) Did you falsely think you were going into labor at any time during the pregnancy? What was that phone call with the doctor/experience like?

I experienced some slight Braxton-Hicks contractions, but I was working a physically demanding job, doing twelve-hour shifts, and just assumed I strained something when lifting or moving. I never had to call my provider for a false alarm.

5) Can you describe how you went into labor and the steps from when you thought you were going into labor until you had your baby in your arms?

My son was a stubborn, breech baby throughout my whole pregnancy. We attempted to flip him by undergoing an external cephalic version (ECV) at thirty-eight weeks so I could have a vaginal delivery. Unfortunately, it was unsuccessful, and I was scheduled for a cesarean section. After having the unsuccessful ECV, I knew that the C-section was our only option to safely get our son out. I feel like half of me was nervous because I was about to undergo a major surgery, and the other half was feeling fine because C-sections are performed every day. Since I work in the medical field, I unfortunately have seen complications that have occurred to women that I was nervous about, but I was hopeful that everything was going to go smoothly. I did have to have the scary but important conversation with my husband about what to do if there were any complications during surgery. We discussed my wishes if something were to go wrong that I had to be put on a ventilator, if it came down to the decision of saving me or the baby, as well as who to call if difficult medical decisions had to be made and he needed support. When preparing for a baby, these aren't things that you want to think about because it is an exciting time for all. But working in the medical field, I have seen too many times that people don't have these conversations with their partners, and then they don't have any idea what to do. It made me feel better going into surgery, knowing that my husband and I had the tough conversation ahead of time to be prepared just in case.

My C-section was scheduled a week after the ECV on December 14, 2021. At around 11:00 p.m. on December 11, I was lying in bed, and my water broke. Now let's talk underprepared when it comes to this lovely part of the journey...definitely not like what you see in the movies! At this point, my midwife and doctor hadn't even talked to me about my water breaking for whatever reason. I was lying in bed and immediately thought I had just peed a little from coughing...embarrassing, but it happens at that stage in the game! Once I made it into the bathroom, I realized it was a slow leak happening every few minutes and began to google what was happening...of course! I'm not sure if I was trying to convince myself that I was in labor at that point. So I called the hospital, and they said I needed to get to the hospital immediately. Upon arrival, I was feeling fine, minus the leaking, so after seeing my vitals and consulting with the on-call provider, they scheduled me for a C-section the next morning at 9:00 a.m. unless conditions were to change overnight. They kept me in the hospital because I was in active labor with a breeched baby. I was having very mild contractions that I didn't even recognize, but they wanted me to stay in case things progressed, and they needed to take me to surgery right away.

The labor and delivery operating room was on the same floor as our overnight room. My husband was allowed to come into the operating room during my surgery once I was prepped and got to sit by my head throughout the procedure. Once our son was out and checked over, they brought him over to us since I was still open on the table so we could meet him. The nurses took our baby into the room next door to get checked out and get all his measurements. I told my husband to go with him while they finished putting me back together. Once my surgery was complete, I was moved back into my hospital bed and wheeled next door into the recovery room with my family where my son and I were able to skin-to-skin contact for about an hour while we were both monitored for any delayed complications. After that, we were taken back to our overnight room and were greeted by our OB nurses that were there to help facilitate feedings and keep checking on me for any complications. I went into surgery on December 12 at 9:00 a.m., and my little man was brought into the world at 9:28 a.m.

6) Can you describe your postdelivery experience at the hospital? Please include your experience with breastfeeding, your body's experience in postdelivery feelings, what the nurses helped with and where you wish they supported you

more, where your baby was, and how long you stayed at the hospital.

We stayed two nights in the hospital after delivery. Our son was in the room with my husband and me the whole time, except when he had to go for testing (hearing, reaction, blood work, etc.) with the nurse to the nursery. The nurse at the time didn't really give us an option to have any testing done in the room. She came in late one evening and said that he needed to go for his hearing test, and she would have him back soon. He was only taken from us for those common tests and for his circumcision. Otherwise, he was in our room for our whole stay.

Breastfeeding was a struggle from the beginning. I did not attend any classes during my pregnancy and only had information that I had gathered from my own research. My son never wanted to latch directly to me. I felt very frustrated because I didn't feel like the nurses or lactation consultant were super helpful. They basically threw a nipple shield on my boob and shoved my son's face at it. I didn't get any guidance on different breastfeeding positions that might be helpful or tips to get him to latch naturally. At this point, my epidural still hadn't worn off from surgery, and I was still loopy from anesthesia, so I wasn't processing everything to the best of my ability. The breastfeeding process felt rushed with little to no direction.

I was sore from surgery once my anesthesia wore off and struggled getting comfortable in the bed, especially trying to find a good breastfeeding position. I also didn't realize after a C-section that I would have such intense vaginal bleeding.

That was never mentioned until it was happening, so it came as a bit of a shock when I finally got to go to the bathroom on my own. I logically know the process and that bleeding would occur, but for whatever reason, seeing a red toilet was a complete shock. Leaving the hospital, I felt great! I felt stiff but didn't have any major pain. I refused a wheelchair and walked out with my family. It felt so good to be up and moving out of the hospital bed!

I had one follow-up a few days after leaving the hospital with the lactation consultant but felt that it was more a checkup for my son to make sure he was gaining weight rather than checking his latch or the mechanics of breastfeeding. She asked me how I was but didn't really have much to say when I was bringing up the struggles we were facing. We had a very difficult time getting my son to latch directly. We ended up using a nipple shield, per the lactation consultant, which was a hassle to maneuver, that and everything else for a good position. She didn't have much input or demonstration, which would have been helpful, to guide us to something that would work best in our situation. I ended up researching different shields and ways to get it to stay in place, as well as how to wean the baby off the shield and even the best positions for larger chested women. After a few short weeks, I became an exclusive pumper and stopped attempting to nurse because the frustrations of positioning and not latching without a shield weren't good for any of us.

7) Can you describe your physical recovery experience at home and how long you worked to recover to "normal"

(i.e., did you go to PT, need X-rays, use advice from parents, wing it, do research into how to recover, etc.)?

From working in the medical field, I knew how important it was to keep moving and stay ahead of any pain during my recovery. Once home, I realized that my "good" pain meds were wearing off and that I was more sore than I had felt leaving the hospital. Moving around at home made me aware all the muscles that had been cut and how I'd taken them for granted on a good day! I didn't have to do any PT or go for X-rays. I did go to the chiropractor before, during, and after my pregnancy, which I think helped keep everything loose. I took advice from the What to Expect mom blogs and lightly from family members.

The biggest part of my postpartum journey that I wasn't prepared for was the postpartum depression and anxiety. I have often heard of women getting the "baby blues" as our bodies try to regulate our hormones and get back to "normal." I honestly believe that providers should do more screening for PPD and let moms know that it's okay to not feel okay! My midwife asked me if I was feeling depressed or anxious at every postpartum appointment, but my answer was always "Of course, I am! I have a newborn and haven't slept in days. I don't know what day it is!" I feel like the conversation ended with some giggles and was never looked into further. I truly believe I should have been put on some medication for anxiety and depression after having my son and think it could have helped immensely. I was not strong enough or comfortable enough to bring it up at my appointments or ask for more help because mental health has such a stigma, and as a new mom, I felt like I needed to have it all together, for some reason.

I can say that my son is recently eighteen months old, and I have just now begun to start feeling like myself again. I can confidently say now that I am around eighteen months postpartum that if I get pregnant again, I will not be shy to ask my doctor for help and not be embarrassed to prioritize my mental health. I started seeing a therapist to help work through many of my PPD issues, and my body is starting to feel like mine again. Recovery, both physically and mentally, was a much longer process than I expected, and I found that it was very much like a grieving process for me.

8) Is there anything else you would like to tell me about your pregnancy?

I contribute a lot of my PPD/PPA to many things that were outside factors not directly related to my pregnancy. I did have a Nexplanon birth control implant placed around twelve weeks postpartum, which I researched that many women have reported increased anxiety and depression with that. I got that removed a few months after stopping breastfeeding and definitely noticed a change in my mental status, but I was also seeing a therapist as well and working through things.

I'm thankful that I was able to find answers and comfort in testimonies from other women going through the same processes but disheartened that it was from strangers on the Internet instead of my network of health providers. Our bodies are made to do such an amazing process that we should feel adequately prepared to start and go through the entire journey. My pregnancy journey was nerve-racking, wonderful, confusing, and amazingly fulfilling all at the same time, giving me the greatest gift, my son.

Mom 4

1) What·were your expectations on pregnancy and the process before going to your first doctor's appointment? Were you happy with the care you received, or did you feel like you weren't properly prepared for what to expect throughout the process?

First pregnancy: When I first got a positive pregnancy test, I was so thrilled. I immediately called my doctor and set up an appointment. I knew that they wouldn't see me until at least eight weeks but didn't realize how long it would feel to wait four weeks to be seen! I remember being so worried that something was going to happen between finding out I was pregnant and going to that first appointment. I just kept taking pregnancy tests every few days because that felt like all I could do to make sure everything was okay. When I went to my first appointment, I expected to walk in and for the doctor to sit down and go over what to expect during pregnancy and appointments. The nurse came in and checked my blood pressure, asked me some questions, sent me for blood work, and then said, "Okay, what questions do you have?" I was taken by surprise! I remember thinking, *I've never been pregnant before! I don't even know what questions*

107

I'm supposed to have! When the doctor came in, he did a transvaginal ultrasound and located the heartbeat. He was concerned that it might be an interstitial pregnancy (a type of ectopic pregnancy), so he called the high-risk doctor for me to be seen the next day. He could tell that I was on the verge of tears, so he tried to reassure me that he didn't think there was an issue but that he wanted to just double-check. I appreciated that he wanted to be thorough and am thankful there wasn't any issue. Overall, I was satisfied with the care I received but definitely felt the responsibility of seeking information was on me.

Second pregnancy: I was much more prepared for pregnancy the second time around! However, even with my prior experience with my firstborn, I was just as anxious!

2) Did you feel like your concerns were adequately heard or did you feel like anything you brought up was always pushed off in a "you're pregnant you're going to be uncomfortable" category?

First and second pregnancy: I always felt that the doctors listened and took my concerns seriously. With that said, I experienced some frustration during both my pregnancies with false labor and receiving guidance from the doctors that I felt could have been helpful.

3) What was your birthing plan before you went to the hospital and how did it differ from what you experienced?

First pregnancy: I didn't have a formal birth plan for this pregnancy. I knew I wanted an epidural and that I wanted to try different positions while I was pushing to prevent tearing. I was definitely not mentally prepared for a C-section.

Second pregnancy: Because I had already had a C-section and because I knew I needed to have my fallopian tubes removed (for unrelated health reasons), I chose to have a C-section for my second delivery. I was much better-prepared because I knew what to expect.

4) Did you falsely think you were going into labor at any time during the pregnancy? What was that phone call with the doctor/experience like?

First pregnancy: With my first pregnancy, I started having contractions around thirty-four weeks. They lasted around a minute and would recur every two to three minutes and last eight to twelve hours. They weren't incredibly strong but were uncomfortable enough that I couldn't sleep through them. Because I had been told that I should call the doctor if I ever experienced contractions that met these criteria, I called the doctor. The first time this happened, I called the doctor in the morning, and he told me to come in that morning to get checked out. I was one-centimeter dilated and 80 percent effaced (at thirty-four weeks). The doctor said I wasn't in labor but that it seemed likely that I'd go into labor early. As a result, he sent me to the hospital for steroid shots to help the baby's lungs to develop more quickly, in case I ended up having him early. As the weeks went on, I continued having these contractions that would last for hours at a consistent rate. Each time I would call the doctor, I'd come in, and they'd check to see if I was in labor and if I was dilating. It seemed like I was just slowly dilating over time. By the time I actually went into labor at thirty-eight weeks and four days, I was already five centimeters, and most of that had occurred during the weeks prior!

Second pregnancy: With my second pregnancy, I experienced the same thing. However, this time, I felt that the doctors weren't as concerned as they had been the first go around. Similarly, I started having contractions weeks before my due date, but when I called the doctor after hours, the response was "Well, if you think you are in labor, you should go to the hospital. Otherwise, you can call and make an appointment in the morning, if you are concerned."

I remember feeling like I wasn't sure if I was supposed to be concerned. During my first pregnancy, they wanted to see me and check that everything was okay. This time, they seemed like they thought this was no big deal. But at the same time, I knew I was following the recommendation to call after experiencing contractions that lasted a minute, every five minutes, that went on for at least two hours. I would even wait until it had been eight or more hours, knowing that I wasn't actually in labor. But when I'd call the doctors, they would say things like "Lay down for a little bit and drink some water. It's probably just Braxton-Hicks." I would tell them that I was lying down because I was sleeping when they started, and they were regular (unlike Braxton-Hicks). I've already had forty-eight ounces of water, and they haven't stopped for hours. I would always get the same response, "Well, if you think you are in labor, go to the hospital. Otherwise, make an appointment in the morning."

Once, when I went to an appointment the morning after a night filled with contractions, I explained everything that I was experiencing, and the doctor said, "Well, you're not in active labor." I remember my eyes burning because I was so frustrated and was trying not to cry. I knew I wasn't in labor. I didn't go to the doctor because I thought I was in labor. I already had a baby. I knew what it felt like to be in labor. I went to the doctor because I didn't understand why I was having regular, consistent contractions for hours and hours. I went to the doctor because when I'd experienced the same thing in my previous pregnancy, the doctors were concerned that I'd go into labor early, and I assumed the concern remained the same for this pregnancy.

In all my internet searches and conversations with doctors, I could never find any information about contractions like these that were clearly different from Braxton-Hicks and lead to dilation but didn't progress into active labor.

5) Can you describe how you went into labor and the steps from when you thought you were going into labor until you had your baby in your arms?

First pregnancy: When I got to the hospital (Sunday around 6:00 p.m.), I was about five centimeters and 100 percent effaced. At that point, my contractions slowed down. They gave me an epidural before giving me Pitocin and breaking my water. It took until about 6:00 a.m. the following morning for me to reach ten centimeters. At that point, I started pushing. I didn't feel pain, but I felt a lot of pressure on my rectum. The epidural was strong enough to take away the pain, but I still had use of my legs. I was able to get in a squatting position while I pushed. However, I wasn't strong enough to hold myself up and maintain that position for very long. The most comfortable position for me was on my hands and knees.

After nearly three hours of pushing, the doctor said I could keep pushing if I wanted but that it was unlikely he was going to come out. Each time I pushed, the baby's heart rate dropped, so she was concerned that the cord was around his neck (which we later learned it was).

At that point, we decided to move forward with the cesarean. Shortly after making that decision, my pain medication wore off. They couldn't give me anything yet because I was getting ready for surgery. So for about thirty minutes, I went from feeling zero pain to feeling the height of labor pains. I also had not mentally prepared for a C-section, so I was an emotional mess. I was terrified about having surgery, and I didn't know exactly what was happening as they wheeled me through the L&D unit.

When I entered the OR and the anesthesiologist administered more of the epidural medication, it numbed my entire body from below my chin to my feet. Most alarmingly, I was unable to swallow. In the panicked state I was in, I started to feel like I was going to die from choking on my saliva, so I just kept turning my head and spitting. (Later, I learned that I was able to swallow but that the numbing made it so that I was unable to feel that I was swallowing. Regardless, it was really terrifying.) The surgery itself was pretty quick, and I was relieved to hear my son's first cries (around 10:00 a.m.).

Right after that, the anesthesiologist said he could offer me something that would allow me to relax and give me some rest. I said yes, and then I don't remember anything else until I got into the recovery room. Accepting whatever the anesthesia was offered is one of my biggest regrets because it made me incredibly groggy for the next twenty-four plus hours. I remember very little from the first day of my son's life, and that is something I've mourned.

I was thirty-eight weeks and four days when he was born. I learned afterward that the reason he was having difficulty coming out was that his head was having trouble clearing my pelvis.

Second pregnancy: Even though the C-section was scheduled a week prior to my due date, I went into labor before my scheduled delivery. After having contractions all night, I went to the doctor the following morning; they confirmed I was about four centimeters and was in labor and sent me to the hospital since I was planning to have a C-section.

When I got to the hospital (around 10:00 a.m.), they told me the OR wouldn't be available until around 3:00 p.m.; however, as they monitored my contractions, they realized they probably wouldn't be able to wait that long. I ended up having the procedure around 1:00 p.m., and our son was delivered shortly after.

During surgery, there was a laceration to my bladder. As a result, I had to wait in the OR for a urologist to come check things out. The urologist wasn't on-site, so we had to wait for him to arrive. What should have been a thirty- to forty-five-minute surgery ended up being around two and a half hours. I wasn't worried while I waited to be stitched up but was disappointed to have to wait two hours to hold my son. My understanding is that this complication during C-sections isn't unheard of but also isn't incredibly common.

6) Can you describe your postdelivery experience at the hospital? Please include your experience with breastfeeding, your body's experience in postdelivery feelings, what the nurses helped with and where you wish they supported you more, where your baby was, and how long you stayed at the hospital.

First pregnancy: I arrived at the hospital on a Sunday night, my son was born on a Monday morning, and we went home on Thursday afternoon (four nights in total—three were postpartum). I was incredibly groggy after surgery. I was constantly falling asleep in the middle of conversations and was afraid I was going to fall asleep while holding or feeding my baby. I also struggled with some depression and anxiety in the first few weeks after he was born.

While at the hospital, I felt fine during the day but really struggled with feeling alone and afraid at night. I was terrified that something would happen to my son, so I hardly slept. During the day, we had lots of visitors, and nurses came in often to check in on me and the baby. But at night, it was dark and quiet. My husband was trying to sleep, and the nurses came in but less frequently. I wanted to sleep but couldn't. I was convinced that if I wasn't always watching our baby, he was going to die. Every noise he made (and newborns make *lots* of noises) startled me, and I would check on him. I felt very alone in my feelings and didn't know how to express them. I wasn't prepared for how emotional I would be postpartum.

Breastfeeding was difficult with my first. He had a really hard time latching. Each nursing session would be around forty-five minutes, and most of that was him crying and me frustratingly trying to get him to latch. I remember my friend being in the room while he was trying to eat, and she could tell I was getting upset, so she asked what she could do to help. She ended up grabbing my breast and trying to put it in his mouth like it were a hamburger, something we laughed about later. The lactation consultants weren't very helpful on this matter. They recognized that he was having difficulty but couldn't pinpoint any reason and didn't have many suggestions. They did give me a nipple shield to try, which was helpful in getting him to latch for the first couple weeks.

The biggest concern was that by the time we left the hospital, he had lost 13 percent of his weight and was struggling to gain it back. As we were leaving the hospital, the lactation consultant came back in one last time to check in. She said, "Yeah, I'm not very impressed with his sucking." But then she didn't have anything else to say! She left the room, and I just started crying. Thankfully, a nurse came in at that moment and I told her everything. I told her I was worried because he wasn't eating well, and we were about to go home, and I didn't know how to make sure he was getting enough. She comforted me and asked me if I wanted to take some formula home just in case. I graciously accepted it. I was surprised that it took about four days for my milk to come in. I felt more relieved once I could visibly feel that he was draining the breast. Even still, he had difficulty with nursing for months. I would pump after every other nursing session and would supplement each feeding with an ounce or two of the expressed milk. It was worth it to ensure he was eating but was exhausting!

Second pregnancy: Because I knew how things had gone the first time around, I made a point to talk with friends and family prior to having our second son about visiting me in the hospital. One of my friends came to see me every day I was in the hospital, just to keep me company. My husband especially appreciated this because it gave him an opportunity to get out of the room without having to worry about me.being lonely since I struggled with feeling depressed and anxious when I was alone. We stayed in the hospital three nights.

Breastfeeding the second time around was much easier. I'm not sure if it was just because I knew what I was doing or if it was because my second son just had an easier time latching. It easily could've been a combination of both! I was always suspicious that we created a problem for our first son by supplementing with expressed milk because he was struggling with nursing, and then we were giving him the bottle so frequently I worried that we were confusing him. However, it was necessary for his weight gain. Doctors were always suggesting maybe I just didn't have enough milk, but that was never the issue. I would pump between eight to twelve ounces in ten minutes! In fact, with my second son, I ended up donating a lot of milk to the milk bank because I ran out of room in my chest freezer! Between donations to the milk bank and another mom who was in need, I donated over one thousand ounces of milk during the first six months of my second son's life. I'm grateful to have been able to do that!

7) Can you describe your physical recovery experience at home and how long you worked to recover to "normal" (i.e., did you go to PT, need X-rays, use advice from parents, wing it, do research into how to recover, etc.)?

First pregnancy: I was very hesitant to walk and do a whole lot after surgery, out of fear. I think that slowed down my recovery a lot. It took about three weeks before I felt somewhat normal, but each week, I felt better and better. I just followed the advice of the nurses and doctors and limited stairs, monitored how much I was bleeding, drank lots of water, tried not to lift much, etc. I have a small umbilical hernia from my first pregnancy and had some separation of my abdomen from both pregnancies (diastasis recti). The hernia has not posed any problems, so I have not had it repaired.

Second pregnancy: Recovery was much harder this time. Surprisingly, I found that recovery from surgery was much less painful the second time around; however, I don't know if that was just a result of there being other factors that complicated my recovery. Because my bladder was nicked during surgery, I had to keep a catheter in for two weeks. That was incredibly uncomfortable. It caused me pain when I slept, and it was difficult to walk, shower, lie down, or sit comfortably with it strapped to my leg. I was also terrified I might get an infection. Occasionally, very small blood clots would pass through the tubing and bag, and I was always worried that it was a sign something was wrong. Thankfully, everything was fine.

I had to have an X-ray after two weeks to make sure my bladder had healed properly. At that time, they were able to remove the catheter. About two days after we came home from the hospital, I got one of the worst migraines I've ever had. Knowing that this could be a sign of postpartum preeclampsia, I called my doctor, and she had me come back to the hospital. This was really hard because I had to decide if I was going to bring my newborn back to the hospital and expose him to all those germs or if I was going to leave him home and be away from him. I ended up leaving him, but after about an hour of being in the hospital and crying from being away from my baby, my husband brought him to me. We waited in triage at the labor and delivery unit. They determined it wasn't preeclampsia but wanted to do a CT scan just to make sure there weren't any neurological issues. The doctor (the same OB who delivered both my boys) was incredibly accommodating while we waited; knowing that we didn't want to take the baby out of L&D, she allowed us to stay in there instead of going to the ER to wait for an available room. Everything was fine, I was given some migraine medication, and we ended up going home.

That night, I tested positive for COVID-19. It turned out the migraine was just the first symptom. I was terrified of what would happen if my baby, who was barely a week old, caught COVID-19. Initially, I had to isolate from my son, which was awful. The only times I could hold him were when I was nursing him. A couple days later, my husband tested positive, at which point we realized that isolating was no longer an option. We both just wore masks and tried not to worry (although, honestly, I did worry). Thankfully, my dad came and stayed with us during that time and helped take care of household tasks and caring for our two-year-old.

8) Is there anything else you would like to tell me about your pregnancy?

I have always been an anxious person, but my anxiety during pregnancy and postpartum skyrocketed. I found my anxiety was the highest during pregnancy and during the first couple months postpartum. Overtime, as hormones began to level out, I could tell that my anxiety was also leveling out. During pregnancy, particularly my first, I worried about the safety of the baby but also about how I'd be as a mom. I was worried that I wouldn't be a good enough mom for my son, whom I already loved so much. I would be up at night crying, worried that I wouldn't be able to give my baby everything he needed. I started seeing a therapist when I was pregnant with my second child because I knew that my anxiety had been so high while I was pregnant with my first. Therapy has definitely helped. I mentioned my anxiety to my OB, but it never seemed to register high enough on their rating scales. Looking back, I wish I could have shared the specifics of my anxiety with my doctor, just to know whether or not what I was experiencing was normal.

My anxiety and emotions were much more under control after my second son was born than they were after my first. When I first came home from the hospital with my firstborn, I was so worried that he would die if we weren't watching him at all hours of the day/night. As a result, my husband and I did shift work for the first two weeks. I was with our son from 8:00 a.m. to 8:00 p.m., and my husband was watching him from 8:00 p.m. to 8:00 a.m. and would wake me up when it was time to feed him. This was really not a sustainable way to live. But I wasn't able to sleep if my firstborn was in the room with me because I would end up watching him, out of fear. So while this was not the best long-term solution, it felt necessary because I knew I needed to sleep, and I knew I wouldn't be able to if someone wasn't watching him.

There were lots of things that really spiked my anxiety with a newborn. Cleanliness and safety were the two biggest things. I was very anxious about bacteria getting in his bottles and making him sick. I would wash and sanitize all bottles and pump parts after every use even though the CDC recommends sanitizing only once a day. I was worried about his car seat straps being tight enough and would get out of the car to double-check them multiple times before we'd leave to go anywhere. If I left milk sitting out one minute longer than the recommended time, I would throw it out. If I had a glass of wine, I would use alcohol test strips to check to see if the milk was safe. And about half the time, even though the strip would be clear, I would doubt the accuracy of the test and would throw out the milk anyway.

While all the anxiety was exhausting and wearing me down, it felt necessary to take extra steps to ensure the safety of my children. I would think, *Washing and sanitizing these parts for the third time today is so annoying, but it's worth it because I can ensure that my child's milk will be safe.* I knew that if I didn't do all these things, I would lay awake at night worried about it. It felt like if I didn't do everything I could to protect my child, even to the point of absurdity, that if anything were to happen to him, it would have been my fault. While my logical brain can say *"that's not true,"* my anxiety was telling me otherwise.

Mom 5

1) What were your expectations on pregnancy and the process before going to your first doctor's appointment? Were you happy with the care you received, or did you feel like you weren't properly prepared for what to expect throughout the process?

First to third pregnancies: I had three miscarriages before having my first baby. My first pregnancy, I had my first OB appointment eight weeks after my positive pregnancy test; they ran blood work to confirm the pregnancy and did a Doppler to attempt to hear a heartbeat (even though a majority of the time, you can't hear a heartbeat this early). Everything looked good, and they had me come back at ten/eleven weeks to do a transvaginal ultrasound; that was when they saw the baby no longer had a heartbeat and had stopped growing at nine and half weeks. The doctor thought oral medicine wouldn't work to naturally remove the baby since the baby was so large, so they recommended a D&C (dilation and curettage). I was very close with my OB and had been seeing her since fifteen, so I trusted her. She recommended we do genetic testing on our baby after the D&C to see if there was anything that was causing the miscarriages and put us at risk for future miscarriages. The doctor called me directly with the results of the genetic testing. The results showed the baby had Turner's syndrome, which is a common genetic condition that can cause a miscarriage. We were told we didn't have any more risk than anyone else would for future pregnancy's and to keep trying. My second and third pregnancies were chemical pregnancies; I lost the baby shortly after having a positive pregnancy test, and they were passed naturally.

Fourth pregnancy: Because of the previous miscarriages and heartache, when I found out I was pregnant with our first daughter, I felt like my husband and I were robbed of the true excitement of finding out we were pregnant. We were so excited and happy, but we were so fearful of another failed pregnancy. The difference with our first daughter, because of the miscarriages, was my doctor referred us to a fertility doctor to monitor early care. I was told to call the fertility office the day I received a positive pregnancy test, and I was able to go in to my fertility OB the next day to get a blood test and to start on vaginal progesterone. I ended up being happy with my care because I felt like I was being monitored closely due to my history, and they were watching the baby attentively. The fertility doctors didn't know what had caused my miscarriages since they'd run tests on me and hadn't found anything, but they decided to try progesterone. They didn't know if low levels were what was causing miscarriages, but they said the progesterone would be a safety net and couldn't hurt anything.

After that initial appointment, I went back forty-eight hours later for another blood draw to make sure my progesterone levels were rising appropriately. At six weeks, I received an ultrasound to confirm the baby had a heartbeat. Two weeks later, at eight weeks, I had another ultrasound to confirm the heartbeat again. Because this was during COVID-19, my husband could not go into these appointments with me, so I was alone and fearful of bad news, which was terrifying. I had my husband come with me to my appointments and sit in the car and wait, so if there was any bad news, I would have him close by. Once everything was confirmed to be progressing well at nine weeks, I was transferred from the fertility clinic my OB had me going to back to my OB. After my first appointment with the OB, I also started seeing a high-risk specialist as well to ensure everything was progressing properly. At ten weeks, they did early blood work for genetic testing since the D&C had Turner's syndrome, and all tests were normal.

Fifth pregnancy: The start of this pregnancy was exactly the same as my first daughter's except my OB was able to do the fertility care since nothing was ever found to be wrong with me. Once I was at the eight- or nine-week mark, we started having trips to the high-risk specialist again. We were still nervous that we might potentially lose the baby, but we were a little more cautiously optimistic and excited for our pregnancy since we'd already had our first daughter.

2) Did you feel like your concerns were adequately heard or did you feel like anything you brought up was always pushed off in a "you're pregnant you're going to be uncomfortable" category?

Fourth pregnancy: The only time I felt like my symptoms were pushed off was when I had pubic symphysis diastasis (PSD). There would be nights I'd be crying trying to stand up because the pain was so bad. Instead of looking at how they could help me, the doctors told me this can happen. It wasn't ignored, but they classified it as "normal" and wrote it off. I know now I could have been getting physical therapy during my pregnancy to help lessen the pain or I could have worn hip binders to help hold my hips together better.

Fifth pregnancy: My PSD was better with my second daughter because I knew what to do to help with the pain. This pregnancy, my high-risk doctor focused a lot on my connective tissue disorder, Ehlers-Danlos syndrome (EDS). I have the hypermobility type of EDS, but there is also a cardiovascular type that is more serious during pregnancy. As a precaution, the doctor sent me for an echocardiogram to make sure there weren't any cardiac concerns.

3) What was your birthing plan before you went to the hospital and how did it differ from what you experienced?

Fourth pregnancy: I did not do, or want, a birthing plan. I have a pediatric nursing background and know how quickly those plans can go out of the window, so I didn't want the added stress of knowing things didn't go as planned. I knew I wanted to try to hold out as long as I could before getting an epidural but was planning to get one. I wanted a vaginal birth but was aware a C-section could happen. My mom had an emergency C-section, and I was nervous it might be hereditary, but luckily, I was able to deliver safely vaginally.

Fifth pregnancy: I also didn't have a birth plan with my second daughter. The only difference from my previous delivery was I asked to use a mirror during delivery so I could see what was going on when I pushed. The doctor delivering my first daughter pulled the mirror out during delivery since she thought I'd want to see my daughter being born, and I liked having it, so I wanted to make sure I had it again to watch my second daughter's delivery.

4) Did you falsely think you were going into labor at any time during the pregnancy? What was that phone call with the doctor/experience like?

Fourth pregnancy: I never thought I went into labor with my first daughter before I actually did. I had the classic water break a couple days before her due date. When we arrived at the hospital, my contractions started.

Fifth pregnancy: For our second daughter, I had been in labor for three days before I knew I was actually in labor. On a Thursday, I noticed some bloody show throughout the day, and around 6:00 p.m., I started having what felt like moderate period cramps. I let it go on until the evening before calling the doctor on call around 9:00 or 10:00 p.m., but I felt like the doctor on call didn't help much. It was clear she had been asleep when I called, and when I was telling her my symptoms, she asked if there were timeable contractions, and there weren't, but I was having timeable pain anywhere from five minutes to twenty minutes. The doctor said it sounded like false labor and to look for a gush, timeable contractions or intensifying pain, and if I had any of those symptoms, I should go to the hospital. The cramping went on all night but cleared up in the morning and were only happening once an hour. Because it was a weekday, I called the office during the day to touch base and tell them what my night was like.

The next night, I started having the same period cramps again around 5:00 p.m., but they were more painful this time. This time, I was up all night long and timing the contractions throughout the night. When I called the doctor, she told me it was still probably false labor since it was clearing up during the day, and hormone levels are higher at night.

By the third day, the cramping started even earlier in the day, and there was no gush, but there had been some fluid that was slowly leaking out. I thought maybe my mucus plug was starting to fall out. I was refusing to call the doctor again since I thought they'd tell me the exact same thing. My husband managed to convince me to call the doctor though, and so I did. This time, there was a new doctor on call, and since there was some fluid with the other symptoms, the doctor had me come in to be safe, especially since we're an hour away from the hospital, and my OB hadn't checked me for dilation the week before at my appointment. The doctor on call still thought it was false labor but wanted to have me come in and get checked out since it was a Saturday, and the office wasn't open to go in and get checked out during the day. So we called my in-laws to watch our daughter and packed a bag even though we thought we'd be home and went to the hospital. We got there around 10:30 p.m. and checked into triage. They determined my water had broken with a litmus test.

5) Can you describe how you went into labor and the steps from when you thought you were going into labor until you had your baby in your arms?

Fourth pregnancy: I had gone to the doctor for my check-in appointment on Thursday, and the doctor didn't think I'd make it through the weekend, so we made an appointment for Monday as a backup but didn't think we'd need it. They were calling for a snowstorm, so on Sunday morning, before the snow got really bad, we went to stay at my grandparents' house since they live five minutes from the hospital. We figured, worst case, we'd at least be close to our appointment on Monday. We packed as if we were going to the hospital, went to my grandparents, and were there all day.

Around 8:30 p.m., I felt like something popped inside me and went into the bathroom, and a large gush of fluid came out. I sat there for a while until it stopped, and then I went and called my husband. I was sitting there, talking to him, when another gush came out. We called the on-call line, and the doctor told us to come into the hospital. Because of the time of night, we went in through the ER. Our first daughter was a COVID-19 baby, so we had to have a mask on from the second we walked into the hospital until we left.

I walked in feeling completely fine and waited for my husband to park before they took us to labor and delivery (L&D). We went up to L&D triage and confirmed my water broke; the doctor came and talked to me in triage to say we should get settled into our room in L&D and she'd come see us when she was done delivering a baby that was ready.

We went to L&D; they set up and got ready for the delivery. They checked for dilation, and I was at three centimeters. They told me to let them know when I wanted an epidural and that it could take some time for an anesthesiologist to show up. I progressed until about 1:00 or 2:00 a.m., and by then, I was getting ready to throw up I was in so much pain. I told my husband it hadn't been that long, so I was worried they'd think I was a wuss for wanting the epidural that quickly. When the nurse came in to checked, I was at eight or nine centimeters, so I needed to get the epidural immediately or I wouldn't be able to get one.

With the epidural, I could still feel everything on my left side. The nurses kept turning me on my left side to see if they could get the epidural to take on that side. The pain eventually subsided, but I could still feel pressure on the left side. I couldn't move or feel my legs at all, so my husband and a nurse were holding them. I pushed for about fifty minutes and had my daughter around 5:00 a.m. The doctor put my daughter on my chest while I was getting stitches, then after the doctor was done, they took her to get her weight and assess her, all in the same room, before giving her back slightly wiped off with a diaper and swaddle. They then left us alone for a little to have some time with our daughter.

Fifth pregnancy (from triage story in question 4): This time, we delivered with the hospital doctor on call. Our doctor was out on family leave, so the week it was her rotation, they'd use the hospital doctor, not someone from our office. I was disappointed that I would have someone I didn't know delivering our baby, but the nurse in triage told me that was the best doctor they had and who she'd want to deliver her baby, so it made me feel a little better.

They thought my amniotic sac wasn't fully ruptured, that there was a small leak, and that's why I didn't see a gush of fluid coming out. The doctor suggested getting an epidural right away, and once it took effect, she would fully rupture the membrane, and things would probably happen pretty quickly at that point. I was ready for the anesthesiologist pretty quickly; maybe an hour later, the nurses made sure the epidural was working and called the doctor in. When she checked my membrane, she saw I was already fully ruptured. The doctor asked when I first called and thought I had been in labor since Thursday when I first started the bloody show.

Thankfully, there were no signs of infection, which is something doctors worry about around forty-eight hours after your water has broken. Since there was no sign of infection, I wasn't put on any antibiotics.

There was no change in dilation between when I came in and when the doctor checked for the rupture. Since the doctor thought my water had broken three days earlier, they didn't want delivery to take a long time, so they started me on a low dose of Pitocin. For this epidural, I could move my toes and legs and still feel everything. I didn't feel pain but could feel the sensations. The doctor said that was okay as long as I didn't feel pain. About an hour after the epidural, I was at ten centimeters and ready to push even though I didn't feel the need to push with this epidural. This delivery was very quick! I only had to push two cycles (three rounds of ten second pushes each) before our daughter was born. After delivery, they immediately put my daughter on my chest and let her stay with us for an hour and a half before they came back to clean her off.

6) Can you describe your post delivery experience at the hospital? Please include your experience with breastfeeding, your body's experience in post delivery, feelings, what the nurses helped with and where you wish they supported you more, where your baby was, and how long you stayed at the hospital.

Fourth pregnancy: In the delivery room, the nurses tried to get me to go to the bathroom. I had an epidural, so I couldn't feel my legs initially, but they got me into a wheelchair so I could try to go to the bathroom. I was able to pee and was feeling okay, so they let us go to the mother-baby unit.

Once we were over there, they were checking on me and my daughter frequently. I was a pediatric nurse with some background in lactation support, so I felt like I knew what to do better for breastfeeding than the average first-time mom, but we immediately asked for the lactation consultant to come to our room while I tried to latch my daughter.

Before the lactation consultant came, she latched right away and was a very powerful sucker. The nurse looked to see if she could help before the lactation consultant came in, but since the latch was good, I didn't get much help or information because my daughter did so well.

I didn't think the hospital lactation consultant was very helpful. I felt like they came in with some photos, and they only told me things I'd known already. They only looked at what I was doing and tried to show me with photos what to do; they didn't try to be hands on and assist me. They told me how to massage the breast to bring the milk down but told me to massage it using a lot of pressure. When I went to my pediatrician's office and talked to the lactation consultant there, she said not to do that, that I could damage a duct. I saw a second lactation consultant before I left the hospital that was better than the first, but I still felt like it was very generic info and photo information more than hands-on help.

In the hospital, I was in a decent amount of pain after delivery. I wasn't comfortable in bed since there was a lot of swelling and lower back pain. I kept stretching and having my husband rub my back a lot. It hurt to get up and go to the bathroom because moving my body hurt. I looked at my stitches pretty soon after birth so I could have a comparison over the next couple days (I suppose this is the nursing side of me). The nurses mostly left us alone besides the check-in points for mom and baby.

The only time our daughter was away from us was when they took her to get testing and then offered to take her to the nursery for two hours that night. When they took her to the nursery, the cleaning staff was in the room beside us, and it was really loud, so we couldn't sleep, so we told the nurse we'd rather have our daughter in our room, and she brought her back. I didn't sleep the entire time, from when I went into labor until we were discharged, so Sunday to Tuesday morning.

By choice, I didn't want to put my baby down; I just wanted to hold her a lot. It wasn't due to anxiety or worry; I just wanted to hold the baby I had waited so long for. We got a twenty-four-hour discharge, which is pretty rare for first-time moms, but because the baby and I were doing so well and the staff felt like I was comfortable, they allowed it.

By the time we were discharged, I was extremely tired after being up for seventy-two hours. The mother-baby nurse was really good at helping us out and made sure we had everything we needed and then some before we left.

Fifth pregnancy: This L&D nurse tried to get me to pee right after delivery as well, but this time, I couldn't. They let me go to recovery without peeing and gave me an hour to pee before they'd have to catheterize me; thankfully, I didn't need the catheter. The lactation consultant experience was the same as with my first daughter, but this time, I really had to flange my daughter's lips to get her to suck, but there were no overall issues. The lactation consultant again told me very generic things, but I felt confident in knowing what I was doing. I had only been not breastfeeding for seven months at this point since I breastfed my oldest until she was seventeen months. It felt like the hospital had to check a box and say a lactation consultant was provided more than they actually wanted to support me in breastfeeding. I didn't sleep at the hospital again. My daughter was in the room with us the whole time except for her PKU test. I didn't want to put her down so I held her most of the time, again not due to worry or anxiety but I just wanted to love on her as much as I could. I physically felt a lot better compared to the first delivery. I didn't want to sit in the bed and was moving around the room since staying still made me feel antsy. We thankfully didn't have to wear our masks much in the recovery unit. If no one was in the room, we didn't have to wear it.

7) Can you describe your physical recovery experience at home and how long you worked to recover to "normal" (i.e., did you go to PT, need X-rays, use advice from parents, wing it, do research into how to recover, etc.)?

Fourth pregnancy: I was in a lot of pain at home; things didn't feel comfortable. Shortly after getting home from the hospital, I started to feel sick, like I had the flu (body aches, feverish, lots of sweating, and was generally feeling awful). I was worried I had picked something up in the hospital and could possibly get my newborn sick.

133

I called my doctor, and she said it sounded like a virus. It was rough feeling sick on top of the pain/discomfort from just giving birth. My daughter happen to have a weight check appointment, and I mentioned it to her pediatrician, and she told me it sounded like I had "milk fever."

She explained it's flu-like symptoms you develop as your milk is coming in. I had never heard of that before, but after a few days, my milk fully came in, and the symptoms subsided. I also had pubic bone separation that continued after birth, so there was pain when I would walk and often clicking.

I felt like it took forever just for me to be able to go out the front doorsteps. I tried not to do steps very often, but we live in a townhouse, so I didn't have too many options.

I was seven to ten days postdelivery when I had excessive bleeding. It happened three times before I called the doctor. My doctor immediately had me come to the office to be evaluated. I was nervous because after the D&C, I had a similar episode and thought that was happening again because the bleeding occurred in the same time frame it had after the D&C. They did blood work to see if I was anemic and a transvaginal ultrasound to see if there were placenta fragments in my uterus they'd have to remove. The doctors determined my uterus had relaxed for a few days and then started contracting again, so there were a lot of clots that needed to get out once it started contracting again. They gave me Cytotec to get my uterus to contract and flush things out to help with the bleeding.

At this appointment, it was also determined my stitches had come out, and they couldn't put them back in at that point, so I had to use Neosporin to help the incision close. They said it wouldn't make anything heal differently; it might just be a cosmetic issue they could fix later if I wanted. Thankfully, everything healed appropriately, and I did not have issues cosmetically.

When I went back for the six-week appointment, I told them I was still having pelvic pain and a lot of pelvic clicking, and they told me that can linger for a while since it's hormone-driven, but it should improve some. I also brought up when I walk, cough, sneeze, or bend down, it felt like something was pushing out of my vagina. The doctor said I had two prolapses, but they were minor, so she wouldn't have brought them up if I hadn't had symptoms and that they would heal with time. I asked about physical therapy, and the doctor said she didn't think I needed it, but she could give me a prescription for it if I wanted to use it later. I decided I wanted to be evaluated by PT, so I called right away to make an appointment.

When I called the PT, there was a six- to eight-week waiting period. At the time, I was upset because I thought if a PT script had been given to me earlier in the pregnancy, when I first complained there was pain, I'd have been able to get in to see the PT right after birth or a little before when I made it in.

When I went to PT, they confirmed the two prolapses, pubic bone separation, abdominal separation, and vaginal muscle tone issues. PT taught me lots of excises to help improve these diagnoses. I even had to have internal vaginal PT because I was experiencing pain with intercourse. It was thought the position my daughter was in in utero had put pressure on the left side of my body since they could feel there was a difference in the muscle tone from the left and right side of my vagina. When I'd go to PT, I'd get vaginal massages, and they'd have me do Kegels to strengthen the vaginal wall. It took about a year for intercourse to feel normal again postpartum. I was in PT for six to eight months before I was discharged. When I was discharged, my prolapse was gone, my pelvic pain improved, vaginal pain with intercourse was mostly gone, and my abdominal separation was gone, but I was frustrated because I still had restrictions. PT was good to bring me back to a general baseline, but it didn't take into account my prepregnancy fitness level. The gap wasn't bridged to get me back to my "normal."

After I was discharged, I emailed my PT to asked for a scaled workout plan to get back to normal and was told there's nothing like that. I asked when I could go back to jumping rope, jumping jacks, and push-ups and was told if I did those again, there was a high chance the pain would come back, and my body could breakdown again. I cried reading the email because nine or ten months postpartum, I was being told I couldn't do what I considered very basic things. Working out was my "me time" and something I always enjoyed, and I was being told I couldn't do that anymore. I was frustrated because I knew Olympians have had babies and can safely get back to an intense workout level, so why couldn't I? I had been very discouraged, wondering if I'd ever get back to normal and be able to do things I enjoyed doing.

I talked to a friend who recommended a health PT who specialized in fitness and athletic postpartum. I thought this is exactly what I needed, but unfortunately, I lived too far from her location, so I messaged her on Instagram, and she responded, telling me she was sorry I'd gotten that information and that it's a common misconception you can't bridge the gap. She taught me how to assess myself at home and recommended an exercise program to help gradually increase the intensity of my workouts. After about three months of her program, I was able to return back to my normal gym routine.

The other issue I experienced postpartum was extreme insomnia. Even when the baby was asleep, I couldn't sleep, so there were lots of tearful days where I was overly exhausted but wouldn't be able to sleep. I was so frustrated with myself. No matter what I did, I couldn't sleep, and I knew I needed sleep. I didn't take melatonin because I was breastfeeding, but I tried Benadryl, and it didn't do anything for me. I had continuous problems sleeping until I stopped breastfeeding at seventeen months. I think it was hormonal because I didn't have a problem before or after breastfeeding with sleep, and it wasn't anxiety or being worried that kept me awake. I just couldn't sleep and would lay there and cry out of frustration. The whole first year of my daughter's life, I probably got two to three hours of sleep, five nights a week, and would have normal rest the other two nights.

Fifth pregnancy: Because it took me so long to recover after my first pregnancy, I was really cautious of not carrying more than ten pounds. I wouldn't even carry the baby in the car seat, and I wouldn't pick up our older daughter because I didn't want to have the bleeding happen again. During my first pregnancy, my uterus did relax, but I also think I was doing too much right after delivery. So this time, I wouldn't do steps more than I had to and would have my husband go and get things during the day if I needed something that wasn't on the floor I was on. This time, I was able to come outside more quickly, and I didn't have as much pelvic pain during or after delivery, which was nice.

When I went in for my six-week appointment, I requested to be evaluated for all this issues I had with my first daughter and get a PT referral immediately. The doctor evaluated me and told me I had a two-finger ab separation, but nothing else—no prolapse, no vaginal pain or vaginal muscle tone issues! She said she didn't think I needed PT, so she wouldn't give me a referral and told me to work with a personal trainer and do all the old things I was given from PT for my first baby.

By the time I hit my six-week appointment, this time, I already recovered to what it took me nine to ten months to recover from after PT the first time. I started doing a gradual postpartum workout and didn't end up going to PT because I felt like I could do it myself.

I'm currently five months postdelivery, and I feel like I'm mostly back to normal, but I'm being cautious with core work and jumping. While I'm not fully back yet, I feel significantly better than before. I do my own assessment every few weeks and follow the plan I'd been doing after my first baby. With this pregnancy, I also developed "milk fever," but I knew what to expect this time. It lasted about two days, and then I felt much better. So far, I haven't experienced any insomnia issues. Of course, there have been sleepless night with having a new baby, and I'm breastfeeding, but I haven't experienced anything like I did with my first daughter.

8) Is there anything else you would like to tell me about your pregnancy?

Becoming a mom is the absolute best! My mom always said you don't know what love is until you have a baby. I never realized how true that was until I was holding my babies in my arms. It is a love like no other. Being a mom is amazing, but it is hard. I learned how important it is to be supported and how to communicate with my husband since we are a team in this parent thing. I learned that it's important to be open and honest about how I was feeling and how I needed to ask for support.

Since I was breastfeeding, there wasn't a whole lot that my husband physically could do. I found myself getting frustrated especially in those earlier weeks where I was up every two hours feeding the baby, and he would be sleeping even though I knew he couldn't do anything. It was me who needed to feed the baby. I wanted him to be there with me in those sleepless nights, to be living in the trenches of parenthood with me. I felt alone and needed support.

After telling him how I felt, we came up with a plan: my husband would get up and change our baby's diaper and get her ready to be fed while I changed my pads and cleaned myself up and went to the bathroom. Then when I was feeding her, he'd fill my ice water back up and make sure I had everything I needed. It was helpful to not feel alone and feel like he was there with me and being supportive. Motherhood can feel lonely and isolating at times, and for me, I especially felt that way with breastfeeding, so having someone who I felt was there for me made it much easier.

Some days, it feels like there's never a reason, or any time, to ungrung and look put together. Most mornings, you're running around, making sure the kids are taken care of, so you don't take the time to put on anything besides yoga pants and a nursing tank top, and by the time you look at the clock again, it's already late afternoon and not worth changing. You get stuck in a rut of feeling like you're not looking the best and wanting to find a reason to look nice or spend time getting dressed in something that isn't yoga pants and a tank top. Taking the little moments for myself helps me be a better mom, whether that's putting on a nice outfit on the weekend so I feel pretty, taking a shower by myself, going to the gym, or even just driving around in the car, listening to music. Being a mom isn't easy, but it's well worth every single struggle, sleepless nights, and tearful moments.

Appendix 3

Baby Registry Recommendations

There are *so many* recommendations on how to build a baby registry online, and my internal conspiracy theorist has a sneaking suspicion that many of them are sponsored by companies because it seems like there are so many things you buy as a first-time parent that you don't actually need. I've put my thoughts on some common baby registry items below. Hopefully, this will help you save money and store less junk in your house:

❖ *Baby clothing*—The cutest baby clothing seems to be the multipiece sets; however, at 2:00 a.m., when your baby poops and pees through their outfit, you are going to want a one piece with a zipper. I'd recommend your newborn clothes be mostly zippered one-pieces. You have so much new going on in your life that you should be constantly doing things to make those first two-ish months a little easier. So make the multiple changes you'll have to do a day a little easier with zippered onesies.

Remember, when adding clothing to the baby registry, your baby will grow significantly faster than you do, so lining up an entire wardrobe for the year in one size isn't recommended. Pay attention to the month your baby will be born in and the weather that time of year, then select clothing size based off the projected weather for that size of your baby X months after delivery.

❖ *Baby clothing—discounted*—This is a little riskier since babies come out at different sizes, but if you're already pressed on money and you don't think you'll have many items purchased off your registry, do the math for what age your baby will be during each season and look at clearance clothes before your baby is due. For example, my son was born in November, so if I was shopping in May and saw the winter baby clothes on clearance, I would buy new-born to six-month-old baby clothing at a discounted rate since I live in the North East, and cold season is usually November to April here. If you're big on the latest fashion, this won't work. If you're big on saving money, it's a good start. Remember, if your baby is born in the summer, they'll still need some long-sleeved onesies since the general rule of thumb after birth is whatever mom and dad are wearing plus one layer of clothing to keep them warm enough.

❖ *Baby gates*—Keep in mind when buying these that your butt has to fit through the baby gate opening, and the higher the bottom ledge, when opened, the more likely you are to trip on them. Baby weight can come off slowly, so holding a squirming baby and trying to wriggle your butt through a too tight space while navigating stairs is danger-ous. I'd go for the less adaptable but wider mouthed gates. Same with tripping. If you're coming up the stairs with a baby in hand and forget there's an additional two-inch step up at the top of your stairs, *wow*, does that hurt your toe. Try to find one that lies flush to the ground.

❖ *Baby monitors*—Spend some good time researching these. There are so many different things people feel they need these for based off their lifestyle that I'm not going to go into recommendations on brands, but keep in mind things like the following:

- Do I want the connection to stretch all the way to my neighbor's house so I can be over there while the baby is sleeping?
- Do I want a Bluetooth connection? Yes, it's nice to be able to log in and see your baby anywhere, but that means the ability to hack them is there as well.
- Do I want a monitor I can view the baby on or just a listening device?
- What is the battery life on the monitor? Will it always need to be connected to a wall, or can I take it around the house with me for two hours and not need to charge it the whole time?

❖ *Baby on Board suction cup sign*—For every car that has a car seat, put a *suction cup* Baby on Board sign on the registry. Why suction cups? These signs serve a purpose, and it's not so people can "drive safer" around you. These signs are there to help emergency responders find your baby if you're in a car accident and the adult(s) in the car are unconscious. So you only put the sign up when the baby is in the car with you, and you put it on the window closest to the car seat. This lets emergency responders, one, know to look for a baby and, two, know what side will get them to the baby faster. If you're driving around town without the baby, take the sign down (hence the suction cups) so an emergency responder isn't risking their life looking for something that isn't there.

❖ *Black Friday*—Try to purchase larger registry items that no one gifted you on deal days: Black Friday, Cyber Monday, Amazon Prime Day, Memorial Day, etc. Some websites even let you set up alerts for when the items will be cheapest. Is it hard to wait sometimes to set up your cute baby space? Absolutely! Can waiting save you a couple hundred dollars? Absolutely!

❖ *Bottle drying racks*—I'm torn on these. The main argument for me is upright drying racks that can sit against a wall and take up less counter space or ones that lay flat on the counter. We have both. The upright one takes up significantly less space, but the prongs to hang things on are larger and end up being able to hold less overall. The flat models that lay on the counter can hold more bottles, and they dry the inside of the bottle better since the bottles are facing straight down instead of hanging at an angle. If you plan to breastfeed and just use the drying rack for the rare bottle and pump parts, I'd recommend the standing drying rack. If you're going to be mostly bottle-feeding, I'd recommend the flat drying rack to allow for the extra material.

❖ *Bottle warmers*—So many registries recommend getting a travel bottle warmer and an at-home bottle warmer. You do not need two. They do the same thing. If you think you'll need a bottle warmer when traveling, just get the traveling one and use it at home the same way you would when you're away and stop taking up so much counter space because it disappears very quickly.

❖ *Changing tables*—I'd highly recommend getting changing tables that have a cleanable surface and do not use fabric covers. When our son was first born, there were some days we went through five changing table covers a day. It added so much extra laundry that we needed to do. Will the cleanable surfaces be a little colder when you put your kid down? Yes, they will. Will they mind? Not in my experience. We had one changing table that used covered fabrics over a washable surface and one that was just the washable plasticky surface, and our son liked the plastic one better. (We think he liked the noise it made when he would move around on it.)

❖ *Diapers*—If you'll be getting your registry items through a baby shower, I'd recommend leaving diapers (and wipes) off your registry and having people bring them as part of a game. For example, if you think we're having a boy, bring diapers; if you think we're having a girl, bring wipes. If you think the baby's name starts with A-M, bring diapers; if you think the baby's name starts with N-Z, bring wipes. It's a fun way to involve your guests while also ensuring you have some good starting materials for when the baby comes.

If you will not be having a baby shower, I'd recommend putting size 1 diapers on the registry and a few of the other sizes up to size 5. In our experience, our baby was so big and grew so fast he was in size 1 diapers almost immediately after he was born and was in size 4 by the time he was six months. If you have a fast-growing baby, you don't need tons of diapers in the smaller sizes, so add more diapers in the large sizes. They'll stay in those sizes longer, and then you can buy the smaller sizes if you need more. Unless you have a massive number of people purchasing things off your registry, you'll have to buy more diapers at some point, so you might as well not have to store unused diapers until/if baby number 2 comes around or end up donating them because your child grew too quickly.

❖ *Gift cards*—You're going to need something that you forgot to get or didn't know you'd need in the few days after your baby is born, and you're not going to feel like running out to get it or chasing it down in a few different stores. Have some form of quick delivery service gift cards available to use in the few days after you get home and need things but don't feel like going out for them. We used Amazon because that's an account we already had.

❖ *Mobile*—I found an incredibly cute mobile that I loved online and was handmade with wood, but the problem was it doesn't move by itself, so my husband and I end up spinning the mobile by hand to calm down our son, which didn't last long. I'd recommend a mobile that will spin itself to save you from constantly needing to respin the mobile.

❖ *Peri bottles*—The hospital gave me two peri bottles. They were nothing fancy at all, but they got the job done. I'd recommend having one bottle per floor and one to keep in the diaper bag since you end up leaving the house sooner than you think you will after delivery. We have three floors, so I had four bottles. Is this an item for mom? Yes. Can it go on the baby registry? Absolutely! You would not need this bottle if you hadn't had a baby.

- *Pump parts and bottles*—Pumps provided by insurance come with one set of pump parts. If you're pumping through the night, make sure you have at least one backup set of pump parts on your baby registry. Saving yourself a nighttime washing of pumps is great for your sleep. If you don't plan on breastfeeding most of the time, I'd make sure you have enough bottles to get through one day without washing them. Remember, as your child grows, so does their appetite, so having small bottles and large bottles on the registry is a good idea. I'd recommend six to eight bottles of each size going on your registry if you plan to exclusively bottle-feed and size 2 bottle nipples (size 1 is usually included with the bottle purchase) since it doesn't take too long for them to size up.

- *Recliner*—On the nights when your baby is sick, and you need to stay up with them most of the night, a comfortable recliner is invaluable! If you want to rest at all when your baby is congested and can't sleep laying down, then a recliner lets you hold them on your chest while also letting you get some sleep in as well. An extra-wide recliner is nice to allow you and baby some space to wiggle around and get more comfortable on a very long uncomfortable night

- *Storage space*—If you don't have a lot of storage space in your house, consider asking for gift cards as part of your registry and explaining they'll be used to buy things like baby gates, JumpaRoos, playpens, high chairs, plates/cups/silverware, etc. that your baby will love, enjoy, and need but cannot use now.

- *Swaddles*—Do yourself a favor and do not get the Velcro swaddles. In my experience, they're much more escapable, and your kid can grow out of them significantly faster than they do a blanket swaddle. For swaddles, think escapable means the baby is awake, so do your best to learn how to swaddle and use blankets. Blankets are softer and can be repurposed for naps and playmats and aren't loud as hell when you undo the swaddle to make it tighter. Imagine having your baby on the brink of sleep, then accidentally having the Velcro stick before you'd finished pulling it tight and having the sound of parting Velcro five inches from your baby's ears…just buy the blankets.

Appendix 4

Hospital Bag Dos and Don'ts

There are a million guides online for hospital bags. I consulted tons of them and had *way* too much packed that I never used, so here is how I will be packing my hospital bag for our second kid. My bag also had our baby's items, so they're included as well:

- ❖ Your own pillow with a unique pillowcase. White pillowcases are what the hospital uses, so this will make sure you get your own pillow back.
- ❖ Two labor dresses that unbutton/unsnap all the way up through the neck.
- ❖ Three to four pairs of underwear.
- ❖ Two robes, two leggings, and two tank tops (nursing tank tops if breastfeeding) for the two to three days you're in the recovery room and the trip home. If you have a C-section, you might want to skip wearing the leggings or roll them down so they do not irritate your incision.
- ❖ Three thick pairs of socks. While my core was hot, my extremities were cold, and the socks at the hospital sucked. If your water breaks while you have socks on, those can get pretty gross, so have extras.
- ❖ Contacts/glasses that you need to get through your time at the hospital.
- ❖ A toothbrush, toothpaste, extra hairbands, and a hairbrush.

❖ Face wash and dry shampoo. The showers at the hospital were tight on space, and it wasn't worth any of the showers I took. Next time, I'll be waiting until I get home to shower and doing the minimum to feel human in between. They have facecloths there you can use to wash your face.

❖ Makeup. It might sound vain, but there were lots of people visiting us and taking pictures, and I wanted to feel good about myself in those photos, so I brought the basics.

❖ A trash bag to put any soiled clothes in to bring home.

❖ One zippered baby onesie in a few relevant sizes (preemie, newborn, or three-month) depending on how your baby was measuring at appointments. You can bring a hat as well if you want a specific one, but the hospital provides hats for the babies to wear.

❖ One set of baby mittens, if your onesie doesn't cover their fingers already. Your baby's nails are *sharp* when they're born, and the hospital recommended we not cut them for a few days, so bring a set of mittens, so when you take your baby home, you can put them in the car and not worry about them scratching themselves while they're not swaddled.

❖ Two or three snack bars. The hospital is pretty stellar about getting you food when you can eat it. These bars are mostly in case there's some form of delay, and you need to eat ASAP.

Things to keep in the car until it's time to go home:

❖ A car seat.

❖ One baby blanket. This is for the car ride home, so leave it in the car seat to clear some space in the room and your bag. The hospital has tons of blankets they use while you're there to swaddle the baby, so you won't need this until you leave.

About the Author

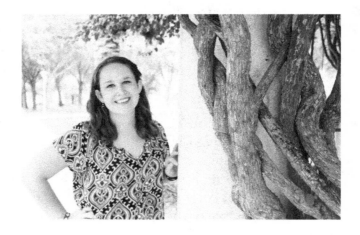

McKenzie Nelson is a first-time mom with a background in engineering. As an engineer, she loves having numbers and peer-reviewed research to back up her decisions. During her pregnancy, she had a hard time finding the type of information she wanted to know readily available. Looking back on her pregnancy, she felt there were so many opportunities to have known what she was heading into but no one to explain what would happen, not doctors, not family, and she didn't have friends who had children already to ask. Her only support was from multiple two-hundred- to seven-hundred-page textbooks she didn't have the time or energy to read.

As a result, she's making her author's debut with a short novella to help moms-to-be struggle less through the first stages of pregnancy and motherhood than she did.

Printed in the USA
CPSIA information can be obtained
at www.ICGtesting.com
LVHW090929270924
792207LV00002B/302

9 798892 211543